A guide to age well and even get younger

Turning 50

149 tips
on how not to grow
Old, **Ugly** and **Dumb**
after a man turns 50

Roger C. DEPETRIS

*This book is dedicated to
everyone turning 50 years old.*

*Small changes in your habits
will improve your health and
well-being.*

Start now. Life is beautiful.

*Happy Birthday.
Roger Claude*

Medical Information

This guidebook is intended to improve the fitness, condition and well-being of 50-year-old men.

These tips are provided for information purposes only and can never replace the recommendations of a health care professional.

With that being said, all readers of this guide should first consult a doctor before embarking on a new fitness journey.

Roger C. DEPETRIS: avoir50ans@gmail.com – www.avoir50ans.com

Advice, Tips and strategy for Men of 50 Years and Over Summary

Page 15 - Introduction

Page 21 - Chapter 1: Assessment, Projects... What to do at 50 years old

The fifties are a wonderful milestone. But how to avoid making the same mistakes as in the past? How can we change things?

10 tips to help you review your past
and start new projects

Page 35 - Chapter 2: How to lower Stress in your Fifties

Stress is a major threat to people's health in their fifties. Its consequences are detrimental when it builds up in the body over time. Our modern lifestyle is to blame for this. But is it the only reason?

10 tips to lower the impact of stress
in your daily life

Page 49 - Chapter 3: How to get quality sleep beyond your fifties

Good sleep is a fundamental component of an active and healthy life. The quality of sleep is built up throughout the day. How and why should you take care of your nights? That is an urgent matter.

13 secrets to better sleep and recover fully
at fifty years of age

Page 65 - Chapter 4: How to improve your fitness after 50 years of age

Your body needs to be kept active in order to function properly. But how do you find the time and motivation to exercise?

10 ideas to easily integrate a physical
activity into your daily routine.

Page 77 - Chapter 5: What to eat after turning 50 years of age

How to eat well? What if eating was nothing more than common sense?

11 simple tips to improve
your eating habits

Page 91 - Chapter 6: How to reinvent yourself and change your habits at 50 years of age

The problem is not that you lack ideas. It's "that you don't do anything WITH these ideas." How do you reinvent yourself and escape a midlife crisis ?

*10 tips to start new habits and
change your life*

Page 105 - Chapter 7: Taking Care of Yourself and Your Appearance at 50 years old

Your appearance is a reflection of the level of your self-confidence. It's time to take action, and start asking yourself the right questions if you are not happy about the current situation.

*10 tips on how to take care of your body
and your appearance*

Page 119 - Chapter 8: Men's Health, Threats in the Fifties

They started showing up at your early 40s. 10 years later, health problems and chronic diseases are on the rise. What can you do about it?

*11 tips to counter daily life threats
and illnesses*

Page 133 - Chapter 9: Sex, Libido, and Testosterone at 50 years of age

Our life as men is very much conditioned by Testosterone. How does this hormone work? Why is it responsible for decreased libido and sexual dysfunction?

11 tips to naturally boost your Testosterone
levels at 50 years of age.

Page 147 - Chapter 10: How to age well after fifty years of age

Is it possible to look 30 years young when you are actually 50 years old? How can you preserve your health and initiate true rejuvenation?

10 tips to reject and stop aging

Page 159 - Chapter 11: A 50-Year-Old Man in his Couple

What's the secret of long-lasting couples? Sharing activities, talking to each other. Happiness is built on little things and tender loving care.

10 tips to commit and strengthen
the bonds of your couple

Page 173 - Chapter 12: Increasing Influential Power in Your Fifties

Increasing your influence and power of persuasion. Friends, family, work... some secrets must be known in order to win affection and to increase our leadership.

10 tips to communicate better and get
more from others

Page 187 - Chapter 13: Professional Life after fifty years

The professional realm is just like a ladder. The more competent you are, the more valuable you become. Acquiring and perfecting new skills appears to be the best solution.

10 tips to become more efficient and
professionally bankable

Page 201 - Chapter 14: Finance and Retirement at your early fifties

What happens when 50 arrives and you have neglected your retirement and finances?

10 tips to reconsider your finances and be better
prepared for retirement

Page 215 - About the author

Page 219 - Resources: List of Useful Links for a
Successful 50th Anniversary Transition

Being 50 years of age

Introduction

Introduction

"Every man has two lives... The second one begins when you realize you only have one."Michel Cymes, Doctor and French Media Person

Health, sleep, stress, food, family, work, finances, projects... This guide includes 14 chapters and covers all aspects of a 50-year-old man's life.

Each chapter provides valuable, easy-to-follow advice. It is also peppered with inspirational quotes and "fun facts". The writing style is simple, easy to read, with lots of resources to help you learn more about the topic.

What to do: You are free to start the guide with any chapter of your choice.

Four basics to get more out of life

«*"Insanity is behaving in the same way and expecting a different result." Albert Einstein, physicist*

Just like an architect, this guide will help you build a solid foundation for the second part of your life. There are four essential pillars to consider when you are 50 years of age:

- *Food*
- *Stress Management*
- *Quality of Sleep*
- *Physical Activity*

Do not seek perfection in just one particular aspect. Rather, strive for the right balance in everything.

What to do: Focus your efforts first on these aspects of your life. Everything else will follow.

The big secret to change everything at 50 years of age

"There's only one way to learn, and that's by taking action."Paulo Coelho, Brazilian novelist

What makes you the man you are today? What defines your health, your finances, your job, your appearance?

The answer to these questions is quite simple. It can be put in two words: **YOUR HABITS**.

Change your habits and your life will follow. It's as simple as that.

This guide is meant to help you do just that.

What to do: Apply these tips as quickly as possible. Don't wait too long!

Chapter 1

Assessment
10 Tips to review your progress and start new projects at 50 years of age

«There's no favorable wind for one who doesn't know where he's going.»Seneca, Roman author and philosopher

The fifties is a wonderful milestone in one's life. But perhaps you feel more pressured as time is running out.

How can we avoid making the same mistakes of the past? What decisions should you make to move forward in life?

How can you turn things around? And why not take on new challenges?

***10 tips to help you evaluate your life
and start new projects.***

1) Looking back at your life and taking things slow

«Success is not about never making mistakes, it's about never making the same mistake twice.» Bernard Shaw, Irish writer

50 years, half a century, time passes so quickly. We even forget to ask ourselves if we are happy.

Stop! Hit the pause button to ponder the different aspects of your life:

Love, Family, Work, Health, Dreams...

What do you like? What should be changed? Looking back on your life to get back on track.

What to do: Looking back takes time, reflection, a pen and a notebook. Plan several 30-minute sessions and write down your answers.

2) Can we change at age 50? What if the mindset is more important than the process?

«The mind is to success what water is to life»
Patrick Louis Richard, French writer

Every change starts with a trigger and an awakening. Then, two key factors follow:

- Choosing a strategy, a method
- Changing your self-image

But why do we often fail? Strategy only accounts for 20% of the final result. It is the mindset that is primarily responsible for success (or failure).

Tip: You can empower your mind with positive affirmations.

More information: "21 Days to Master Affirmations" by Louise Hay

3) Set Goals to better control your present

«A goal is not always meant to be reached, it often serves simply as something to aim at.»Bruce Lee

Goals are often associated with a result to be reached in the future. This is a mistake. No one has control over the future, only present moment matters.

Setting goals brings clarity, enthusiasm and motivation to the present. Not in 2, 5 or 10 years.

Things to think about: Setting goals should keep you active, happy and full of energy. PRESENTLY.

4) The art of setting your Goals to better visualize them

«He who has no goals will never achieve them»
Sun Tzu, Chinese Commander

The brain can visualize and translate goals into reality. But they still need to be well set out.

Example of a good way to express your goals:
I want to climb Mont Blanc before I turn 55. I want to take a picture at the summit and hang it in my living room.

A well-defined goal helps the brain act and plan:
Save money, improve your physical health, hire a professional guide, etc.

What to do: Develop the habit of setting out your goals accurately and vividly.

5) Your Mind: the only weapon to overcome your midlife crisis

«Good things happen to those who hustle»
Anaïs Nin, American author

Your life feels dull. Your work, your family no longer interests you. You are nostalgic. These signs are quite obvious: **you're in for a midlife crisis.**

Existential crisis, losing your bearings... turning 50 means taking a step back.

Asking yourself questions, reflecting, meditating, in order to give meaning to your life on a personal and professional level.

What to do: Go through all the tips in this guide. Ponder on it, talk with the important people in your life.

6) How to deal with challenges at 50 years of age

«*If you can't change a situation that is harming you, you can always choose the attitude you're going to face it with*»
Viktor Frankl, Austrian neurologist and psychiatrist

By the age of 50, you have already overcome many problems, gone through many crises. This ability of the mind to cope with adversity is called resilience.

A strength of character that is forward-looking and forces you to take action so that you don't let yourself get beaten down. Accepting the situation (well), putting things into perspective, taking action... are the first steps to becoming more resilient.

More information: "Resilient: How to Grow an Unshakable Core of Calm, Strength, and Happiness" by Ph.D. Hanson Rick - videos by Jocko Willick

7) How to learn new things in 20 hours, even at 50 years of age

«Forget the 10,000-hour rule... what if you could learn a new skill in 20 hours or less?» Josh Kaufman, American author

Lack of skills is a great obstacle to dreams and ambitions. Lack of time, fear, idleness... all prevent you from learning new things.

However, 20 hours (and a well-organized plan) are enough to acquire the basics of any field.

Josh Kaufman's method breaks down the learning of a new skill into a daily sequence of 45 minutes for a month.

More information: "The First 20 hours, How to Learn Anything Fast" by Josh Kaufman

8) How to be passionate and fascinating as a fifty-year-old

«Every child is an artist, the problem is to remain an artist once he grows up» Pablo Picasso, Spanish painter

How to live an exciting life at 50 years of age? Trust your intuition. Your passions are buried deep within you, and have been there for a very long time. Remember the 10-12 year old boy you once were.

Go to a bookstore, what are you more interested in? Learn new skills, connect and share with others, try new things... **be alive**.

What to do: You can learn new skills online. Many websites (Udemy, Coursera, Skillshare, Rype, Treehouse...) offer a variety of courses on endless topics.

9) Take action, the Universal Law to success

«Practice makes perfect» French proverb

This guide is packed with tips to work on every aspect of your life: Health, Food, Sleep, Work...

But there is no magic bullet. In order to make progress, you need **to put knowledge and theory into action.**

Don't be afraid to make mistakes. Nothing will ever be perfect at first. This is the price to pay to move forward, to change or rebuild your life after fifty years.

More information: "Start With Why: How Great Leaders Inspire Everyone To Take Action" by Simon Sinek.

10) Why make your own bucket list at 50 years of age?

«The tragedy of life is not that it ends so soon. It's that we wait so long to begin it» Unknown author

It's time to spice up your life so that you can live fully.

A bucket list is a list of things you want to accomplish before you move on to the next life.

Drinking a Guinness in Dublin, watching a World Cup match, walking on the Great Wall of China, getting a dog, finding your first love...

Well, you get the idea.

More information: "The List" by Yuval Abramovitz.

Chapter 2

Stress
10 Tips to be more Zen after turning 50 years of age

Fun fact: Stress can make your blood thicker. It is a useful defense mechanism when an injury occurs. It is much less useful when your blood is thick all the time (risk of blood clots, strokes and heart attacks).

The WHO refers to stress as the greatest threat to health. The body's response to an attack is vital in difficult situations, but the consequences of stress are harmful when it lasts in time.

As we're constantly busy, modern life is a major factor in stress-related issues. However, man's behaviour allows more and more stress to creep into his life. And thus having an impact on his health.

10 tips to reduce the impact of stress in your daily life

1) Limit the use of your cell phone in the morning

«Focusing on what's important and leaving out the irrelevant is hard because the whole world seems to be lining up to swamp you with stupid things to do» Tim Ferriss, American author and speaker.

Using your cell phone to wake up is not a good idea. With your cell phone in your hand, you might be tempted to check your email, social media, news... and get your first dose of stress for the day.

Your mind is productive in the morning. Don't waste it! Start with sports, meditation, reading, writing... focus on YOURSELF.

What to do: leave your phone in airplane mode in the morning. Use a regular alarm clock.

2) Start a news diet

«The media acts as a threat amplifier» Jacques Attali,
French writer and economist

Have you ever been on vacation abroad, with no shocking news? How wonderful! News brings up disasters, incidents and illnesses.

This constant flow of negative news increases your stress level.

Think about it: how much control do you have over all the information you receive? None, other than having to put up with it.

What to do: Forget about the news. Turn off news notifications on your cell phone. Try it for a month.

3) Cardiac coherence or how to reduce stress in less than 5 minutes

«Breathing is the way to our inner self»

We breathe more than 20,000 times a day, without actually paying much attention to it. How unfortunate! Breathing synchronizes our autonomic nervous system (ANS).

Much like the control tower at the airport, the ANS is responsible for overseeing *digestion, heartbeat, hormone secretions, blood sugar and stress levels.*

Cardiac coherence exercises focus on breathing through the nose slowly and deeply to reach a rate of 6 breaths per minute.

Within a few minutes of doing these breathing exercises, the parasympathetic nervous system kicks in. The stress level in the body then decreases rapidly.

To do: Easier than meditation, start with 5 minutes of cardiac coherence 3 times a day. It has no side effects and works almost immediately.

4) Get rid of the toxic people around you

«Tell me who your friends are, I'll tell you who you are»
French proverb

Friends, family... we are used to say that we become the people we hang out with. To change for the better and feel more serene, you have to keep your distance from toxic people.

It is not easy. But, just like a black hole, this kind of relationship drains your energy and wears you down mentally. Lighten up and take off.

What to do: Focus your attention on yourself. Don't waste time and energy with the wrong people. Move away from toxic relationships to find peace of mind.

5) The Benefits of Laughter on Stress Levels

Fun fact: A Norwegian study revealed that laughter and a sense of humor could increase life expectancy by up to 7 years.

According to this study, laughter and a sense of humor increase our life span. More surprisingly, we could live longer and healthier.

The release of cortisol, the main stress hormone, decreases when we laugh. But what is laughter?

Having a sense of humor, a witticism... that sparkle in your eyes.

The good news is that a sense of humor can be picked up and developed.

Must Read: "How to Be Funny: The One and Only Practical Guide for Every Occasion, Situation, and Disaster (no kidding)" by Jon Macks.

6) Anxiety, 5 ways to decrease it

«The body loves the attention you give it. This is a very powerful form of self-healing. Most illnesses creep in when you're not in your body» Eckhart Tolle, Writer and Speaker

The concepts of Stress and Anxiety are sometimes confused. Stress is a defense mechanism for the body. Anxiety is a permanent state of worry that wears off gradually.

It is important to manage stress and reduce anxiety. Here's how you can do it:

- **Learn to breathe** properly,
- Eat well,
- Sleep well,
- Disconnect,
- Take magnesium supplements.

What to do: Practice deep abdominal breathing to reduce stress levels.

7) Burnout, relieving your emotional stress to better cope with it

«You can't release tension by keeping your mouth tight, your jaws clenched and locking your fist in your pocket»
Catherine Vasey

1 employee out of 4 had already suffered from a burnout (CEGOS 2015 Survey). The expression "I feel stressed" should be taken as an early warning sign.

Letting this mental strain build up is bad, instead it is more about letting it go:

Jumping, moving, screaming, running, singing... Allow your body to physically get rid of the stress.

Must read: "Peak Performance: Elevate Your Game, Avoid Burnout, and Thrive with the New Science of Success" by Brad Stulberg.

8) Everyone is addicted! When your cell phone becomes a new form of addiction.

Fun fact: According to a British study, we use our phone an average of 221 times per day.

Mail, social media, weather, news... even the fifty-year-olds can't help it, we are constantly checking our cell phone. A phenomenon that isolates each and every one of us in a solitary bubble.

Being constantly connected to the Internet, where each notification interrupts the present moment and adds new doses of stress. This irrepressible need to reply instantly causes us to feel less Zen.

The cell phone is a new form of slavery. But then again, who is the master?

What to do urgently: Cut down your cell phone addiction. You can download on your smartphone some applications to stay focused.

9) Sport and endorphins, a recipe for happiness

«*Motivation is what gets you started. Habit is what keeps you going*» *Jim Rohn, American Writer and Speaker*

Our body releases endorphins during physical effort. This natural hormone has effects similar to those of morphine. Its release by the brain induces a feeling of relaxation and well-being.

Being active, exercising... is therefore good for the body and for mental health. All the more reason to get started (especially after the age of fifty).

What to do: *walk, run, cycle...* start a regular physical activity. Outdoors, it's even better.

10) Organizing, to put order in your life

«Being organized is to refuse to be invaded by chaos and confusion» Olivier Deauville, psychologist and psychiatrist

Reducing stress by taking back control of your life. It's a great plan, but how do you do it after 50 years of age?

Being organized, getting rid of unnecessary things and gaining serenity. It makes sense, because a well-ordered environment provides a sense of security.

Our mothers were right: "Keep your room clean".

Read and apply the recommendations in Marie Kondo's book "The Life-Changing Magic of Tidying Up".

Chapter 3

Sleep
13 Tips for better sleep after turning 50 years of age

"Sleep is the golden chain that ties health and our bodies together." Thomas Dekker - writer

Many men suffer from sleep disorders without ever fully realizing the consequences.

However, quality sleep is the secret to boosting your immune system, balancing your metabolism, giving energy to your brain and extending your life span.

Good sleep is the foundation for an active and healthy life. So take care of your nights. It's quite crucial.

13 tips for better sleep and full recovery after turning 50 years of age

1) Why is sleep important?

«Where care lodges, sleep will never lie»
William Shakespeare in Romeo and Juliet

Professor Satchin Panda compares sleep to his workplace.

When you arrive in the morning, everything seems normal. Yet during the night maintenance crews came in to change the bulbs and fix the breakdowns. Others came to clean up and take out the trash.

Essential repairs to your health are carried out while you sleep.

Tip: At 50 years old, you need at least 7 hours of sleep every night.

2) How do mattresses affect your nights?

Fun fact: Sleeping well is all about proper posture. The best sleeping position is when your spine is straight, flat and on your back.

We spend 1/3 of our lives sleeping. The quality of mattresses is really worth considering.

Antibacterial, fungicide, fireproof ... mattresses are full of chemicals and other endocrine disruptors.

Over time, mattresses tend to lose their form and cannot support our bodies properly anymore. As a result, we wake up in the morning tired and each night a little more intoxicated.

What to do: It is recommended to change mattresses every 10 years. And, why not invest in an ecological mattress free of all harmful substances.

3) Consistency is the key to quality sleep

«The tiger also needs some sleep»
Chinese proverb

According to experts, a 50-year-old man needs to sleep between 7 and 9 hours a night to be in great shape.

Bedtimes and waking hours must follow some kind of a ritual and be consistent.

When needed, a short nap in the afternoon is preferred to oversleeping in the morning.

What to do: Take a shower and finish with cold water before going to bed. It is an excellent natural sleeping aid.

4) No blue light before sleeping

Fun fact: According to experts, the harmful effects of blue light start after 30 minutes of exposure.

We spend on average more than 5 hours in front of the screens (*laptop, computer, television, tablet*). The light emitted by these devices is dangerous for our health.

It leads to an early deterioration of the retina, a predisposition condition to AMD and cataracts.

Exposure to blue light at night interferes with our internal clock. Its radiation blocks the production of hormones needed to fall asleep.

What to do: Make sure to limit your exposure to smartphone and tablet screens at night. Filter, blue light goggles... solutions exist to minimize the risks.

5) When to exercise to get a good quality sleep

«The future belongs to those who get up early»
Henry Gauthier-Villars, French novelist

Exercising at the right time allows the body to be in s sync with its biological cycles.

Ideally, physical exercise should be carried out in the morning and in the open air.

On the other hand, work out in the evening when the body is ready for sleep is not the best thing to do. Sleep well at night and prepare yourself during the day.

What to do: Even for a short time, physical activities in the morning lead to a better quality of sleep.

6) Why you should never keep your mobile in your bedroom

«Everything has its wonders, even darkness and silence.»
Helen Keller, American author and politician.

The bedroom is not just like any other room. Where one keeps browsing the internet, answering emails or sending text messages.

At night in your bed, you disconnect; you rest; you get to find your other half (for couples).

In order to sleep well, you need to turn off your cell phone and put it away in another room of the house.

What to do: In case you need an alarm, buy yourself a classic alarm clock.

7) Get enough sunlight during the day for a good night's sleep

«Sleep is the beginning of our day, not the end»
Satchin Panda, researcher in biological rhythm

The key to a good sleep is to be exposed to natural light during the day and darkness at night.

This seems obvious, but according to one study: sleep is more profound, more restorative, when we expose ourselves to natural sunlight.

Walk your dog, go for a walk... get into the habit of going outdoors every day.

What to do: Getting the morning sunlight on your skin is very beneficial. You can use phototherapy lamp to get your daily dose of light, especially in the winter.

8) Learn how to connect with the Earth to improve your life.

«In the universe, everything is energy, everything is vibration, from the infinitely small to the infinitely large...»
Albert Einstein, Nobel Prize in Physics in 1921

Put your shoes back on! That's what we often tell our kids. Big mistake. Grounding is about reconnecting the body with the Earth's natural energy.

It reduces inflammation and stress, improves the quality of sleep...

Earth energy is beneficial for health and sleep. Taking control over your health requires simple actions. You would be surprised to know all the benefits of Grounding.

Must read: "Earthing: The Most Important Health Discovery Ever" by Dr. Stephen T. Sinatra, M.D.

9) How to reduce snoring and sleep apnea

Did you know: Why do you wake up in the morning with a dry mouth? It's because you breathe through your mouth while you sleep.

When you watch a baby sleep, the first thing you notice is how calm and serene he or she is. Breathing is slow and mostly through the nose.

Unfortunately, things change with age. By the age of 50, most men have trouble breathing during the day. And even worse during the night. In many cases, breathing remains shallow, rapid and is done through the mouth.

Waking up at night because you are thirsty, or waking up in the morning with a dry mouth, snoring and sleep apnea, these disorders are all signs of bad breathing.

Over 50 years of age, it is important to learn to breathe properly again. FYI, there are small devices to tape your lips during the night (see myotape).

To do: for a good night's sleep, practice 5 to 10 minutes of deep breathing through the nose in the evening before going to sleep.Example: *breathe in on 4 beats and breathe out on 8 beats.*

10) Sleeping well requires absolute darkness

Fun fact: Your skin has sensors that are sensitive to light. In the presence of light, these sensors send messages to the brain which then affect sleep.

The brain needs darkness to release the hormones that are essential for falling asleep. Light sources are picked up by the eyes, even when the eyelids are closed.

Similarly, exposure to bright light should be reduced before bedtime. And even more so, that of screens (laptop, tablet...) which can disrupt the functioning of the brain.

What to do: Get rid of all light sources in your room and invest in blackout curtains.

11) Make love not war

«Improving sleep would be an ideal solution for better health»
Institut National du Sommeil et de Vigilance (INSV)

Here is another important thing you can do in your bedroom: Make love.

Before going to sleep, it can be a powerful sedative:

Endorphin, Dopamine, Melatonin, Prolactin, Oxytocin, the orgasm releases all these hormones for relaxation and falling asleep.

What to do: No comment!

12) No alcohol before falling asleep

*«Drugs caused 100 deaths last year, alcohol fifty thousand.
Choose your side, comrade» Coluche, French
Humorist and Actor 1944 - 1986*

You fall asleep quickly, heavily, when you are drunk. However, the presence of alcohol in the body leads to poor quality sleep.

Alcohol interferes with the hormonal system and the mechanisms of long and short-term memory.

This is why we sometimes experience memory blackouts in the morning after an entire evening of drinking.

What to do: Don't drink alcohol before going to bed for a few hours at least, or have an aperitif at noon to give yourself time to digest.

13) The power of the 10-minute nap

Fun fact: The word siesta comes from the Latin "sixta" which means "the sixth hour of the day".

A nap is great for fixing bad night's sleep.

This short break allows the body and mind to recover from fatigue, to think better and to recharge the batteries.

According to an Australian study: **10 minutes** would be the optimal nap time.

Ideally, it should take place in the afternoon, between 2 and 3 pm.

More information: "Take a Nap! Change Your Life" by Sara Mednick.

Chapter 4

Sports
10 Tips for getting back into physical activity at 50 years of age

Fun fact: Physical activity helps our body to purify itself and support our immune system. It is by moving our body, muscle contractions that make the lymph circulate in the lymphatic system.

Just like eating, drinking, sleeping... physical activity, even if it is minimal, needs to be carried out on a regular basis to keep 50-year-old men in good health.

Our body needs to be active in order to function properly. But how do we find the time to work out?

How do we fit daily physical activity into our busy schedules?

10 ideas to easily integrate physical activity into your daily routine.

1) How to get back into sports at 50 years of age?

«What is important is seldom urgent and what is urgent, seldom important» Dwight David Eisenhower, President of the United States

The word sports is quite specific. At 50 years of age, physical activity must be part of daily life in order to keep fit.

Gym, walking, running but also dancing, gardening or yoga everyone has their own preferences.

The secret is to comply with two criteria, **Consistency** and **Frequency**.

15 minutes of daily physical activity is much better than a long weekly session of 2 hours.

Keep in mind: "You're not 20 years old anymore," talk to your doctor before starting any physical activity.

2) The mini trampoline exercise, the ideal solution when you're short of time

Fun fact: Every time you bounce, you are subjected to both weightlessness and extreme gravity. You constantly alternate muscle contraction and relaxation.

Compact, efficient and affordable, the mini trampoline (*around 40 inches diameter*) is ideal for busy people.

Here are **6 reasons** to get hooked on it:

- It uses all 638 muscles of the human body.
- It protects the joints
- It increases your energy level
- It stimulates lymphatic drainage
- It helps you cut down on body fat
- It improves your balance

What to do: One 10-minute session per day for one month. You'll thank me later.

3) Nordic Walking, a complete sport for all year round

Fun fact: Nordic walking uses 90% of muscle mass. The entire body is strengthened: triceps, trapezius, back muscles, lumbar muscles, abdominal muscles, buttocks and thighs.

Nordic walking is a complete sport, and is accessible for everyone.

You use sticks to exercise the arms and relieve the joints.

Nordic walking is enjoyed outdoors all year round.

You will thus enjoy the benefits of natural sunlight. Although in winter, it is anything but luxurious.

Must read: "Complete Guide to Nordic Walking" by Gill Stewart.

4) The Kettlebell: a great plus for weight training

Fun fact: Originally from Russia, Red Army soldiers used kettlebell during training.

The kettlebell is a cast-iron weight, shaped like a cannonball, with a flat bottom and a wide handle.

Through swinging motions, kettlebell exercises strengthen the whole body and increase its power.

Different weights are available. It is a complete tool for gaining mass/muscular strength and for cardio workouts.

What to do: Buy yourself a 12 kg kettlebell and leave it in the trunk of your car. You can then end your walk or jog with a 10-minute workout using the kettlebell.

5) Turn your car into a gym!

«Discipline equals freedom» Jocko Willink, author,
former commander of the Navy Seals

Don't have enough time for sports?

It's not surprising: leaving the house, going to the gym, taking a shower, changing clothes... requires a minimum of 2-3 hours. It's quite demanding.

The solution is to leave in your car: *sneakers, windbreakers, walking sticks, kettlebell...*

You are now ready for a 20-minute workout every day - worry free.

What to do: Choose a consistent daily activity, even if it's for a short period of time, rather than one big workout session every 36th day of the month.

6) The benefits of playing sports outdoors

Fun fact: According to The Telegraph, exercising outdoors makes people twice as happy as going to the gym.

Convenient and inexpensive, lowers blood pressure, helps you lose weight, increases energy, and is good for your morale... There are many benefits to exercising outdoors.

Being surrounded by nature, in the forest, in a park is much better than a contained and air-conditioned atmosphere in a gym.

Running, cycling, Nordic walking... outdoors, even in winter, your body will thank you.

What to do: There are many possibilities for outdoor sports. It's up to you to find the one that suits you the best.

7) The Afghan walk to go the distance and walk for a long time without getting tired

Did you know that? The Afghan walk is a way of breathing that allows you to synchronize your steps with your breathing.

Just like with your car's gearbox, the Afghan walk ensures that you are always at the right "speed".

This practice's base rhythm is done by breathing through the nose and following a cycle of 8 steps: *3 steps when breathing in, 1 pause beat, 3 steps when breathing out and 1 pause beat.*

Depending on how steep the ground is, you can adapt your breathing to extend your breathing when exhaling, or get rid of the pauses... the Afghan walk ensures optimal oxygenation, a perfect balance between oxygen and carbon dioxide.

You will be able to walk longer without getting too tired. This breathing helps to improve your respiratory capacity and to practice a form of meditation while walking. Nothing but bliss and satisfaction.

To do: watch some tutorials on YouTube to learn more about the Afghan walk.

8) The benefits of running

Fun fact: In 2012, three triathletes over 80 years of age finished the Hawaii Ironman at the World Championship event.

Running provides both physical and mental benefits. When you run on a regular basis, it stimulates:

Bone growth, your heart is stronger, you burn fats easier, your cholesterol level is lowered. Running also helps release **endorphins** (happiness hormone).

According to another study: running is much more effective than walking. It also helps with the development of **mitochondria**.

What to do: Talk to your doctor before starting an intensive running activity.

9) Cold showers tone up your blood vessels

Fun fact: Cold showers are an effective sleeping aid.

This is probably the best investment in terms of time/outcome for your health.

Try ending all your showers with 3 minutes of cold (freezing cold) water.

Cold shower benefits for the body are tremendous. Start with your feet, legs and then your forearms.

The secret: Count down in your head from 5 to 0, and then pour the freezing cold water on the rest of your body.

What to do: Cold showers are best when you feel tired, out of shape or hungover.

10) Core strengthening, keeping you fresh and on fire!

«The appearance requires art and finesse; The truth, calm and simplicity» Emmanuel Kant, German Philosopher

At 50 years of age, you have to take care of your physique. Core strengthening exercises are very effective for this matter.

Core strengthening exercise strengthens your spine, boosts your metabolism and helps you look your best.

Try core strengthening exercices on a daily basis. It can be done anywhere and doesn't take much of your time.

Must read: "Diamond-Cut Abs: How to Engineer The Ultimate Six-Pack--Minimalist Methods for Maximal Results" by Danny Kavadlo

Chapter 5

Nutrition
11 Tips on how to eat better after turning 50 years of age

«Let your food be your only medicine»
Hippocrates, Greek philosopher

Choosing food and mealtimes are the basics of a healthy lifestyle.

NIHMR points out that "nutrition is a key factor in the incidence of most chronic diseases".

So how do we eat well? Should we eat organic, become vegetarian or vegan?

What if food was nothing more than common sense?

11 simple tips to improve
your food choices

1) 3 rules to keep a balanced diet

«The doctor of the future will give no medicine but will interest her or his patient in a proper diet and in the cause and prevention of diseases» Thomas Edison
American inventor and scientist

In his book "Mangeons Vrai" Anthony Fardet, a researcher in preventive nutrition, advocates:

1) Include 85% plant-based products in your diet as opposed to 15% animal products.
2) Limit the consumption of ultra-processed products, packed with additives and preservatives (those with more than 5 elements in their composition).
3) Eat more local and seasonal products.

What to do: You don't have to be Paul Bocuse or Gordon Ramsay, just get yourself in the kitchen.

2) At what time should we eat? Complying with the body's biorythm

«I try to manage my day by my circadian rhythms because the creativity is such an elusive thing, and I could easily just stomp over it doing my administrative stuff.
Scott Adams, cartoonist and writer

We focus too much on the food composition, but rarely on **the time we eat**.

Yet eating at any given time offsets our internal clock, which is based on a 24-hour circadian rhythm.

This dysregulation is the trigger for many chronic and inflammatory diseases.

In short, we must avoid eating at night and keep a period **from 12 to 14 hours without having to eat** anything at all (*except drinking water*).

More information: «The Circadian Code: Lose Weight, Supercharge Your Energy, and Transform Your Health from Morning to Midnight» by Satchin Panda PhD.

3) Cleanse and keep your body hydrated every morning

Fun fact: On average, we lose half a liter of water every night.

During the hours of sleep, the body is still functioning and regenerating. The body clears itself of unwanted substances and toxins through the kidneys, digestive system and sweating.

Drinking water in the morning is essential to "cleanse" the body. You then rehydrate your organs and activate your metabolism for the day ahead.

What to do: Try and drink a few large cups of water (*at room temperature*) in the morning as soon as you wake up.

4) Breathing and eating relationship

Did you know? Very ancient human skulls show perfectly aligned teeth. This is no longer the case today with the widespread use of orthodontics among young people.

We chew less and less. On the one hand, we spend less time at the table; on the other hand, our cooked and industrial food is made up of more and more of soft products.

As a result, for many people, chewing is becoming less and less important.

This is not without consequences on the shape of our jaw, on the shape of our face, or the positioning of our tongue.

Eventually, **not chewing affects our airways** and leads to nasal obstruction, which causes snoring, sleep apnea and bad nights.

What to do: introduce raw, hard, non-industrial food into your diet to make you chew more.

5) To remain in shape, avoid fried food

*«Eating fried food in a restaurant is the stupidest thing to do...
It's probably worse than smoking. Because at least nicotine has
benefits» Dave Asprey*

Eating fried foods regularly is harmful to your health.
Fried food contains substances that can damage cells and
blood vessels.

Digesting fried food slows down the body and speeds up
the aging process. The quality of frying oils deteriorates
with usage, thus making fried food even more toxic to the
body.

In short, you should cut back on french fries.

Keep away from: *Chips, French fries, fried chicken and fish,*
especially in restaurants, self-service restaurants, canteens...

6) 3 reasons to cut down on red meat consumption

Fun fact: Dark circles under the eyes, fetid breath, unpleasant body odor, high blood pressure... are red flags. Our digestive system takes a lot of time and effort to digest red meat.

Reducing the consumption of red meat will help you:

1) Preserve the environment: 15,000 liters of water are needed to produce 1 kg of beef meat,
2) Improve your health: red meat increases the risk of diseases such as colon, pancreatic and prostate cancer,
3) Saving animals: every year 65 billion animals are slaughtered.

What to do: Cut down on red meat because now you know why!

7) Sugar and Cancer, best buddies !

«Cancer lives primarily on sugar»
Dr David Servan-Schreiber

Sugar is always part of our diet: white flour, soda, hidden sugar...

We consume an average 35 kg of refined sugar per person per year. The body cannot withstand such a large quantity.

According to Professor David Servan-Schreiber *"Cancer, resulting from the anarchic development of cells, feeds on sugar, which acts as a nutrient helping spread the disease"*.

What to do: Now that you are aware of the effects of sugar, you should start reducing your sugar consumption considerably.

8) Fake sugar, sweetener, light, low-fat... why should you avoid this kind of food?

«Aspartame is a silent poison. As it is used to replace sugar and reduce food's caloric intake, aspartame actually acts the opposite way. It increases chances of developing obesity and diabetes» Henriette Chardak, journalist and author

Sweetened, low-fat products... are a great marketing innovation. Claiming to help promote a healthy diet, it's exactly the opposite that is happening.

To reach their goals, manufacturers use synthetic products and chemical processes.

As a result, our organism is overwhelmed by more and more chemical products. This, in the long run, becomes harmful to our bodies.

Must read: "10 Reasons to Give Up Diet Soda". from health.com

9) 10 Foods you should eat on a regular basis after turning 50 years of age

«Always keep a middle ground in everything you do in life»
Confucius, Chinese philosopher

- Tomato (for antioxidants)
- Oats (for the heart)
- Avocado (omega 3)
- Broccoli (for the bladder, memory)
- Eggs (for muscles)
- Almond (for a flat belly)
- Olive oil, linseed oil (for the brain)
- Salmon (omega 3)
- Dark chocolate (for mood and memory)
- Low-mineral water (for hydration)

Must read: "How Not To Diet: The Groundbreaking Science of Healthy, Permanent Weight Loss" by Michael Greger.

10) Choosing your supplements: the golden rule

Fun fact: 75% of the population has a magnesium deficiency? This is quite alarming as this mineral is involved in more than 300 metabolic reactions in the body.

Food supplements have their pros and cons. However, our diet and lifestyle can't provide us with all the nutrients we need every day.

Supplements are therefore a practical solution to compensate for these deficiencies.

Golden rule: Choose supplements based on natural products. Avoid synthetic products.

Try: Green Superfood supplements by Amazing Grasse or those from Athletic Greens.

11) The 15 hour fast, an easy detox for our body

«Intermittent fasting is essential ... people are less tired, their skin is brighter. There are also fewer risks for developing asthma, allergies, rheumatism and their DNA is strengthened»
Dr Frédéric Saldmann,

Here's a very simple way to help our bodies function better. Intermittent fasting, or fasting for 15 hours, allows our digestive system to take a break.

Basically, it means not eating after 8 pm (*except for drinking water*) and resuming the next day around noon. The therapeutic and purifying virtues of this diet are tremendous.

Must read: "You Are Your Own Best Medicine" by Frédéric Saldmann..

Chapter 6

Habits
10 Tips to reinvent yourself even after turning 50 years of age

«Insanity is behaving in the same way and expecting a different outcome» Albert Einstein

Are you happy with your life? Do you ever feel frustrated, stuck in a life where nothing is happening?

It's not that you lack ideas. It's that you're doing NOTHING with them. So how do you turn your ideas into reality?

The secret to reinventing yourself: Take action, take risks, experiment and explore.

10 tips on how to reinvent yourself and change your life after 50 years of age

1) Going from reflection to action with the 5-second rule

«Just do it» Nike's famous advertising slogan

Before taking action, the brain looks for reasons and excuses for not doing anything. Author Mel Robbins has shown that one simple **countdown** can transform one's life.

By counting backwards (5, 4, 3, 2, 1 Action), the brain goes from thinking mode to action mode.

Simple at first thought, this habit makes it possible to take action and overcome doubts and uncertainties.

Must read: «The 5 Second Rule» by Mel Robbins.

2) Discipline equals freedom

«Discipline is the foundation of all achievement»
Michel Bouthot, author

No wonder this advice was given by a former military man. For Jocko Willink (*former Navy Seals officer*), freedom requires discipline... and knowing how to follow the rules: *get up early, eat well, exercise...*

When you think about it, it's all about discipline, consistency in order to change your habits and be successful.

Must read: «Extreme Ownership» by Jocko Willink.

3) Reconsider your life by sorting out or using the KonMari method.

«Trash cans are the best storage accessories»
Frédéric Dard, writer

What if, before you try and change your life, you start looking all around it. *Clothes, books, papers, objects of sentimental value...* Marie Kondo recommends a method to help you unclutter your life.

Throw, give away, so as to keep only the essentials. And find out who you want to be after turning fifty.

This method calls for introspection by looking back into your past, even though it can be painful at times.

Must read: Tips and advice from Marie Kondo's book "The Life-Changing Magic of Tidying: The Japanese Art".

4) Never stop learning, keep up with your times!

«Life is like riding a bicycle, you have to keep moving forward so you don't lose your balance» Albert Einstein

It goes without saying that the world is constantly changing. When it comes to the professional field, some jobs are disappearing, others are being created.

How can you keep up with your times at 50 years of age?

1) Expand and acquire new skills so that you don't risk being left out.
2) Use your vacation leave for skills training or opt for independent learning.

Remember : **Stalling leads to regression.**

Tips: udemy.com offers more than 100,000 video lessons on almost every topic.

5) The secret to changing your habits: brain neuroplasticity

«Changing your habits leads to changing your life»
Benoît Wojtenka, entrepreneur

The brain often operates in autopilot mode. It does not like the unknown or new things and prefer to stay in the "comfort zone".

Forcing yourself to make changes, especially if you don't like your actual situation, is not easy.

The key to success is to establish new habits in order to replace the old ones. Your brain is malleable, unravel it.

Must read: «The Power of Habit: Why We Do What We Do, and How to Change» by Charles Duhigg.

6) The Miracle of Getting Up Early to Change Your Life

«The future belongs to those who get up early»
Henry Gauthier-Villars, writer

Reading, meditation, reflection, sports... all these activities take time. Which often you don't have, caught up in the hustle and bustle of your days.

The solution is to follow **the Miracle Morning ritual**: Get up around 6 a.m. to practice 6 "Life Savers" activities:

- Silence, Affirmations, Visualization, Exercises, Reading, Writing.

Extreme but effective.

More information: by Hal Elrod «The Miracle Morning: The 6 Habits That Will Transform Your Life Before 8AM».

7) Listening to podcasts, an easy way to grow and develop yourself

«The most important moment is the present, for if you don't take care of your present you might miss your future»
Bernard Werber, The Day of the Ants

There are other ways to learn than by reading. On your way to work, while jogging, in the car... you can listen to podcasts while doing something else.

The topics covered are broad and numerous. Free, accessible through your cell phone. Podcasts are a modern and powerful way to learn.

What to do: Enjoy your daily rides with Apple or Spotify and listen to podcasts on your smartphone about *health, stock market, food, sports, business, learning English and more.*

8) Failure is not an option. Never give up!

«Failure is the foundation of success» Lao-tzu, Chinese sage and contemporary of Confucius

Tips from this guide will help you learn new habits and practices. It won't be easy! And of course, nothing is perfect at first.

Keep trying, fail, do better, but don't give up. Go step by step.

Failure is inevitable and as the saying goes "*Rome was not built in one day*".

Must read: «Shoe Dog: A Memoir by the Creator of NIKE» by Phil Knight. A great lesson of courage, humility and perseverance to build such an empire.

9) Mentors, an inspiration to follow

«The perfect example would be all a father can do for his children» Thomas Mann, Nobel Prize for Literature in 1929

When you were a child, you had your parents as your role models. But now, who inspires you?

To make big changes in your life, you should take advice from people you look up to: **mentors.**

Writers, artists, athletes, celebrities, friends... surround yourself with invaluable advisors.

What to do: Who do you look up to? Find out everything there is to know about these people so that they are familiar to you. Think about what they would do before you make a decision.

10) Visualization, the art of using your imagination to change your life

Fun fact: The effectiveness of a placebo drug can in some cases reach 70%.

The brain doesn't tell the difference between a real or imaginary story. Try feeding your brain great stories.

They will help your brain visualize and create the 50-year-old man you dream of becoming.

The creative power is within each and every one of us. Learn how to develop it by simply using positive affirmations.

Must read: «Techniques Creative Visualization: Use the Power of Your Imagination to Create What You Want in Life» by Shakti Gawain.

Chapter 7

Appearance
10 Tips on how to take care of yourself in your 50's

«Self-confidence is the first key to success»
Ralph Waldo Emerson, American philosopher

After all these years in the service of others, don't you think it's time to take care of yourself? Too busy hustling for your family, career, friends.

What about your appearance? It reflects the level of your self-confidence. It's time to get things done if you're not happy with the current situation. You have to be first comfortable in your body to be comfortable in your mind.

10 tips to increase your self-confidence, take care of your body and your appearance.

1) The secret for a new life and a new beginning

«In life there are no solutions; instead, it's all about creating forces, and solutions follow» Antoine de Saint-Exupéry, French writer, poet and aviator.

Caught up with the daily routine, few people take the time to reflect. Time passes by, gains speed and causes them to lose control.

Serenity consists in taking a break. Asking yourself where are you headed and what you want, establishing crystal clear objectives.

Living in harmony with oneself remains a great challenge for a 50-year-old man.

What to do: Pick up a piece of paper and a pencil every so often and reflect on your life. Refer the Miracle Morning practices in the chapter Reinventing yourself at 50 years of age.

2) The sauna is a great solution for the body and mind of 50-year-old men.

Fun fact: According to a Finnish study*, sauna sessions have a beneficial effect on blood pressure and heart rate.

Taking time for yourself, taking care of your body and mind are valuable moments. The hammams and saunas are the ideal places for this purpose. Saunas help cleanse your body and give you a feeling of well-being.

Almost miraculously, stress decreases after one session and **testosterone levels increase**. Combined with cold baths your body will thank you for it.

What to do: Sauna can be enjoyed all year round. Go regularly for sauna sessions to get rid of mental stress and to cleanse your body.

3) Purifying your body by reducing your exposure to chemicals

Fun fact: Did you know that? A WWF study identified the presence of 73 chemicals that are harmful to health in the blood of members of the European community.

How do you keep yourself safe from the chemicals that are poisoning your body? Well, you can start in your own bathroom.

Personal hygiene products, care products, are loaded with substances that are harmful to health (*paraben, endocrine disruptors and other allergens ...*).

Get rid of them and go for natural products, for soap, and you'll do just fine.

Tip: Try coconut oil for your skin care.

4) Update your wardrobe to celebrate half a century

«Clothes and manners do not make the man; but when he is made, they greatly improve his appearance» Arthur Ashe

Strangely enough, January's sales have just started as we are writing these lines. Sales or not, go to H&M, Zara, Uniclo... and update your wardrobe.

Bring the new you into line.

Tip: At 50, avoid clothes that would make you look old (velvet, quilted) and don't fall for things that would make you look younger.

More information: "The Handbook of Style: A Man's Guide to Looking Good" by "Esquire Magazine".

5) How to cut down on alcohol in your fifties

Fun fact: Alcohol increases the effects of aromatase. Aromatase is an enzyme that converts Testosterone into Estrogen.

Sometimes we just feel the need for a drink. Then one glass leads to a second glass, and so on. The trick is to always go for water first.

You shouldn't drink alcohol to quench your thirst. Start with a few glasses of water. Then, switch between alcohol and water.

Drink alcohol only to enjoy the taste, the pleasure and keep your alcohol consumption to a minimum.

What to do: Before a party or an aperitif, try to drink half a liter of water. Caution, alcohol consumption comes with risks; make sure to follow this guide to cut down on your drinking.

6) Cold showers, this simple ritual can transform your life.

Fun fact: Finland has more than 200 winter swimming clubs. Every year, 150,000 Finns swim in the icy waters of lakes and inlets.

Cold temperatures are extremely beneficial to the body: it reduces body fat, improves tonicity, immunity and blood circulation, and it's good for stress and sleep.

In order to get the most out of it, try finishing you shower with cold freezing water. First the feet and legs, then the entire body.

What to do: Kneipp cures in Germany, cryotherapy in France, cold showers... All of these solutions will provide your body with great benefits.

7) Taking care of your feet

Fun fact: Feet are connected to all the other organs of the body by more than 7,000 nerve endings.

Unpleasant odors, itching, infections, fungus... feet are often overlooked and neglected. Yet they require daily attention in order to remain in good condition and healthy.

Feet must be:

- Regularly moisturized (coconut oil, Nigel oil),
- Well dried to avoid fungus,
- Protected by wearing proper footwear.

They also require be nice socks for extra class.

Tip: How can you treat stubborn toenail fungus? For beautiful and healthy feet, use a combination of lemon juice and aspirin.

8) Cider vinegar every morning, the new formula for well-being

Fun fact: For those who do not like the taste, cider vinegar capsules are now available.

Drinking water in the morning is essential to keep the body hydrated. You can add two tablespoons of cider vinegar to start your day:

It helps with weight loss, lowers blood pressure and it's good for your skin... Just like Tim Ferriss suggests, cider vinegar has many benefits for your health.

Tip: Choose an organic and unfiltered cider vinegar (such as Bragg). Note: Cider vinegar should not replace your entire breakfast.

9) Good bowel movement, it's all about the position!

Fun fact: In France, screening for colorectal cancer after 50 years of age has been standard practice since 2009.

We always talk about food and the importance of a healthy diet. But we rarely talk about how to properly go for a number two: going for a poop.

Modern toilets are convenient. However, the position in which we sit is not adapted to our physiology.

In order to fix this, simply lift up your knees to adjust the inclination of your pelvis. This posture is much better for a good bowel movement.

Tip: You can put your feet on the toilet waste basket. You can also use a stool specially adapted for this purpose (see squattypotty).

10) Taking care of your intestines, your other brain

Fun fact: Your intestines are 8 meters long and contain no less than 100,000 billion bacteria. It is called our second brain.

In order to be beautiful on the outside, you have to look after the inside. Your intestine ensures your bowel movement and plays an important role in your emotions.

When maintained in good health, your intestines effectively help eliminate toxins that give you this unhealthy appearance and make you look sick.

And when properly balanced, our intestinal flora positively impacts our weight, skin, hair and even our mood.

Must read: "Gut: The Inside Story of Our Body's Most Underrated Organ" by Giulia Enders.

Chapter 8

Health
11 Tips for Staying
Healthy After Fifty

Did you know that? Most chronic diseases (cancer, cardiovascular disease, hypertension, depression... the list is long) are consequences of our environment and lifestyle.

They pointed the tip of their noses at the dawn of your forties. Ten years later, health problems and chronic diseases are on the rise and must be taken seriously.

A brief overview of the problems that threaten the health, well-being and energy of men in their fifties.

11 Strategies to Combat Health Threats at Age 50

1) Blood, Heart, Hormones: better to take stock at fifty years old

Did you know that? In France, there is a peak in the onset of myocardial infarction during the weekend.

Health problems are insidious. They settle slowly, silently, without being talked about at first.

At the age of 50, it is time to carry out: a blood test, a cardiac test, a hormone test (Testosterone, DHEA...).

Hormones affect how you will age, your sexuality and all aspects of your life.

Do: make an appointment with your general practitioner and ask for a prescription for these tests.

2) Colon cancer or when carelessness can kill

Did you know that? According to the Medical Research Foundation:1 in 30 people will be confronted with colorectal cancer in their lifetime.

Detected in time, colorectal cancer can be cured 9 times out of 10. However, every year in France 18,000 people die from this cancer.

Answer quickly to the invitation to perform a free screening, generalized in France since 2009.

However, caution is still called for, even in the event of a negative result. Polyps that do not bleed are not detected by this test.

Read: «The Definitive Guide to Cancer: An Integrative Approach to Prevention, Treatment, and Healing (Alternative Medicine Guides)» by Lise N. Alschuler.

3) Keep your brain healthy to prevent stroke.

*Did you know that? The walnut looks just like the brain.
Rightly so, with its fatty acids and minerals,
this nut is very good for brain health.*

Facial paralysis, weakness, difficulty speaking, confusion... are signs of stroke. If these symptoms are present, call 112 or 911 immediately.

To keep your brain healthy: Make sure to

- Sleep well, and watch your diet,
- Play sports, stay sexually active,
- Learn continuously,
- Maintain social relationships

In order to stimulate and develop new neurons

Read: "Prevent heart attack and stroke" (French book) by Dr. Michel de Lorgeril.

4) High blood pressure threatens the heart and arteries at age 50.

Did you know that? In 2018, nearly half a million deaths in the United States included hypertension as a primary or contributing cause (cdc.gov).

Headaches, dizziness, the feeling of a fly in front of the eyes... these signs warn of **high blood pressure**, the scourge of modern times.

Treatment with antihypertensive medication must be prescribed. In all cases, make sure:

Control stress, practice regular physical activity, limit alcohol and salt, prohibit smoking,

To help the body fight hypertension naturally.

Do: Avoid eating already prepared food. They are often too fatty, rich in salt and sugar. And buy yourself a cookbook.

5) Diabetes, a real threat

Did you know that? Since 2010, in France the driver's license issued to diabetics is valid for five years.

The need to urinate often, excessive thirst, big appetite but weight loss and lack of energy are warning signs of **diabetes**. This disease is linked to pancreatic failure.

To help this organ get better, say goodbye to junk food. Instead, choose broccoli, cauliflower and Brussels sprouts.

Test: Prepare a juice of Brussels sprouts, carrots and lettuce, ideal to detoxify the pancreas.

6) Bladder leakage, difficult erections, causing by a tired perineum

Did you know that? More than 18 million men in the United States over age 20 are affected by erectile dysfunction.

At age 50, it is common to suffer from bladder weakness and to experience difficult erections.

In both cases, and before you rush into Viagra, you can strengthen and tone your pelvic muscles with appropriate exercises.

This set of muscles forms like a hammock in the lower part of the pelvis.

Do: Kegel exercises, daily series of 10 rapid contractions of the perineum. The results appear after 3 months of practice. you can also do **breathing techniques** to straight your pelvic muscle

7) 6 tips to halt the decline in Testosterone at age 50

Did you know: Paradoxically, it is the decrease of testosterone in our ancestors, 5000 years ago, that allowed the rise of civilization.

Andropause or low testosterone affects men over 40 years of age. This decline leads to a decrease in sexual desire, muscle wasting, a change in mood, fear of risk.

How to fight naturally against andropause:

- Sleep well, reduce sugar,
- Take zinc, practice intermittent fasting,
- Expose yourself to natural light,
- Practice cardio sessions

Do: a cure of food supplements based on zinc and magnesium.

8) 3 tips to keep your prostate healthy

Did you know that? The prostate is a gland the size of a chestnut.

Starting at the age of fifty, two abnormalities threaten the prostate: hypertrophy (enlargement) and, more seriously, cancer.

Professor François Desgrandchamps gives three recommendations for maintaining a healthy prostate:

- Control your diet, beware of bad fats
- Have regular physical activity
- To have a harmonious sex life (at least 20 ejaculations per month)

Test: Take food supplements based on turmeric and pumpkin seeds.

9) Being healthy at 50! A question of rhythm

"Life is about rhythm. We vibrate, our hearts are pumping blood, and we are a rhythm machine, that's what we are."
Mickey Hart, musician

Our organism works according to an internal clock, based on a 24-hour cycle. The synchronization of the rhythm is done thanks to the day/night periods.

Eating anytime, being exposed to blue light in the evening, working at night... disrupt the clock. And have serious consequences on sleep, the immune system, the cardiovascular system, memory, brain...

Read more: «The Body Clock Guide to Better Health: How to Use your Body's Natural Clock to Fight Illness and Achieve Maximum Health» by Michael Smolensky.

10) Circadian Rhythms and Chronic Diseases

In 2017, the Nobel Prize in Medicine is awarded to three researchers for their work on molecular mechanisms and circadian rhythms in humans.

Chronic illnesses, these long-term conditions, are affecting more and more men:

Obesity, diabetes, cardiovascular diseases, hypertension, respiratory diseases, inflammations: They are rarely cured, we live with them.

Experiments have shown the primordial role of circadian rhythms in humans. Respecting the day/night cycle allows our body to function optimally and also to stay healthy.

Read more: Professor Satchin Panda's work on circadian rhythms.

11) Tingling, redness, headaches ... your eyes get tired.

Did you know that? Sight problems increase because of screens and reduced time spent outdoors.

Modern life is not tender with the eyes. Hours glued to screens (*smartphones, computers*) cause stress and eye fatigue.

These symptoms can be alleviated by exercising. The eye gym allows you to maintain mobility, rest and re-educate your eyes.

It doesn't mean avoiding glasses. But we never know.

Read more: "How To Improve Your Vision Naturally: Strategies and Exercises to Restore Your Eyesight" by Nick Stanton..

Chapter 9

Sex
11 Tips to boost your Testosterone and Libido after 50 years old

«As when I was 20 years old, I swallowed the spring
Young, fun, I shine like a new gun
I've got new blood, I want a thousand chicks.»
excerpt from Sonotone, Claude MC Solar

Our lives as men are linked to Testosterone, a hormone made in the testicles. With age, especially after the age of 50, the production of Testosterone tends to decrease.

The consequences are dramatic on the sexual appetite, the quality of erections, the difficulty to ejaculate.

But Testosterone deficiency is not a fatality. It can be avoided or even reversible.

11 tips to naturally support the production of Testosterone in 50-year-old men

1) Decrease in Testosterone, effects that don't stop at sexuality alone.

Did you know that? New research suggests that one out of four men over 30 have low testosterone levels (ABC News)

Are you familiar with the expression "he's gotten old"? The **drop in testosterone** is probably responsible for this.

Its perverse effects can impact you and transform you in 1 or 2 year(s):

- Decreased physical fitness, general fatigue, apathy,
- Low morale, pessimism, anxiety, irritability,
- Lack of sexual desire, erectile dysfunction,
- Muscle breakdown, joint pain, overweight

Do: The blood test is used to measure the Testosterone level. It is very useful to know if you are affected or not. Talk to your doctor.

2) The secret to stopping Testo's decline: working on the fundamentals

Did you know that? Studies have shown that the average Testosterone level in men today is 25% lower than it was in the 1980s.

Magic products to increase your testo do not exist.

Certain plants and minerals promote hormone secretion. But above all, we must consolidate the pillars of a healthy life:

- Diet, sleep, exercise and stress management.

Some studies show that **the increase of porn watching** on the internet and masturbation are also **leading to a decrease in Testosterone levels for men**.

Problems with erections and libido are signs of disturbances in the body. Restart on good bass.

Read and apply the tips in Chapters 2, 3, 4 and 5 of this guide first.

3) Hypopressive breathing for a flat stomach and an improved erection

«He who masters his breathing, masters his life»

Hypopressive breathing or inverted breathing helps you get a flat stomach and better sexual stamina after age 50.

When you breathe in, the diaphragm moves downward and your belly expands. When exhaling, the diaphragm moves up and the belly bulges in. With hypopressive breathing, **we reverse this pattern**. The belly is tucked in when breathing in and expanded when breathing out.

These exercises will strengthen your abdominal muscles, tone up your diaphragm as well as your perineum. By working on the perineum, men recover a better quality of erection. This breathing acts as well on the entire digestive system.

To top it all off, hypopressive breathing also helps with **urinary incontinence**, a problem that affects more and more men after the age of 50.

To do: Try 5 to 10 minutes of hypopressive breathing in the morning when you wake up, on an empty stomach. After a few weeks of practice, you will start to see results.

4) Limit alcohol to stay a Man

«Alcohol can convert Testosterone into Estrogen»
Jed Diamond, author and psychotherapist

Lack of Testosterone makes a man weak, docile and impotent. Alcohol consumption is particularly responsible for this. It exacerbates the female part of the man.

Alcohol promotes the conversion of Testosterone into Estrogen (female sex hormone), through the action of enzymes called aromatases.

Sorry for the beer lover, but this phenomenon is amplified by the hops present in the beer.

Advice: Avoid beer in particular. Limit your consumption to two glasses of alcohol a day. Schedule alcohol-free days to let your liver rest.

5) How to manage your weight and reduce abdominal fat at age 50

Did you know that? It is extremely difficult to lose weight and reduce fat mass with low Testosterone levels.

Overweight, obesity and low testosterone levels are linked. Studies have shown that 40% of overweight people have a Testo deficiency.

The situation is even worse with diabetes, where it is close to 50%. More worrisome, Testosterone deficiency promotes the development of abdominal fat.

You now know where the **overweight** that awaits men at 50 years old comes from.

Do: Lose weight to increase testosterone and decrease estrogen levels.

6) Hormones are produced in the silence of the night.

«Your life does not get better by chance, it gets better by change» Jim Rohn, American writer and philosopher

Why do you wake up with an erection? You should worry if it's no longer the case. Most testosterone is produced during sleep.

After a 7-hour night, Testosterone levels increase by an average of 30%.

Working or watching TV, up to dawn and neglecting your sleep is therefore tantamount to writing off your libido. Wouldn't that be a shame?

Do: A cold shower before going to bed helps you fall asleep. Batteries recharge during sleep.

7) Stress and Testosterone: like water and fire

Did you know that? Men with a waist circumference greater than 40 inches have a high probability of having low testosterone levels.

Why is it hard to think when you're stressed? Again, it's the hormones' fault. Stress increases one hormone: **cortisol**

Testosterone and Cortisol come from the same hormonal blocks. Like communicating vessels when one increases the other decreases and vice versa.

Managing stress is one of the keys to keeping an optimal Testosterone level.

Advice: Practice meditation to better manage your stress.

8) Diet: a precious help to increase testosterone levels

«Health depends more on precautions than on doctors»
Jacques-Bénigne Bossuet, French writer

Two main principles to support the testo through food:

- **Promote good fat**: Testosterone is made mainly from fatty acids (olive oil, avocado, walnuts, hazelnuts, salmon...).
- **Avoid sugar**: Sugar raises insulin and lowers testo levels.

These foods are harmful to the production of Testosterone:

- *Junk food, soy, flax, mint, hops, dairy products, cereals.*

Read more: «The Hormone Solution» by Dr Thierry Hertoghe.

9) Adopt regular physical activity to naturally support testosterone levels.

«When you start something new. You have to walk before you run» Barbara Hannah Grufferman, American health coach

To be in shape, physical activity (walking, cycling, gardening...) must be almost daily. And, gently, if you start exercising again.

But to really enhance Testosterone, rather favour short, high-intensity sports sessions.

Indeed, endurance sports tend to raise cortisol, the stress hormone, which is bad for Testosterone.

Do: Focus on sports such as Cross Fit and HIIT exercises. Always ask your doctor's opinion on the health of your heart.

10) Endocrine disruptors: the enemies of your sexuality

Did you know that? The endocrine system understands: Pituitary, Thyroid, Pancreas, Testicles, Adrenal Glands.

The endocrine system and our hormones are confused by chemical molecules from the modern world.

Walking, airing regularly in the middle of nature, by the sea is highly recommended to get as far away as possible from endocrine disruptors.

Likewise, to avoid a drop in testosterone levels, it should be banned:

- Ultra-transformed food, microwave heating, chemicals in the home,
- Unnatural care and hygiene products, pesticides...

Read more: "Green Enough: Eat Better, Live Cleaner, Be Happier--All Without Driving Your Family Crazy!" by Leah Segedie

11) What food supplements to choose to boost your hormones at 50 years old

Did you know that 20 to 30 minutes of exposure to the sun increases Testo's rate up to 120%.

Testosterone levels must first be supported by a healthy lifestyle:

- *Eat well, sleep well, play sports, manage stress.*

Certain plants and minerals naturally support the Testo level of men after the age of 50:

- ZMA: zinc, magnesium and vitamin B6
- Tribulus Terrestris, a plant known to improve the libido.
- Ashwagandha, the Indian Ginseng
- Maca from Peru

Advise: Choose food supplements of natural origin for better assimilation.

Chapter 10

Aging
10 Tips for Not
Getting Old at 50

«A man becomes old when his regrets take the place of his dreams» John Barrymore, American actor

What is your biological age? Can you, at age 50, be the biological age of a 35-year-old person? Yes, it is possible!

Take care of yourself, adopt good habits... You can change and preserve your health capital.

Organs, hormones, muscles, skin, brain, energy... What are the secrets to true rejuvenation?

10 tips to help your body purify itself, function better and turn back the clock.

1) Keeping your brain in top shape, long live the fat

«Knowing how to listen means possessing, in addition to one's own, the brains of others» Leonardo da Vinci

When you eat, one out of every five bites is used to feed the brain. This energy-consuming, nut-like organ is particularly fond of fat as a source of energy.

Include foods rich in **omega 3** in your diet to keep your brain healthy:

- Oils (flax, rapeseed, walnut, olive),
- Fish (sardines, mackerel, salmon),
- Egg,
- Avocado

Test: A nutritional supplement of omega 3 based on fish oil to boost brain function.

2) How to look young: a question of collagen

«Objects in stores are carefully examined, but when it comes to people, they are judged by their appearance»
Aristippus of Cyrene, Greek philosopher

Having beautiful skin is a sign of success, happiness and health. Collagen is a protein produced by the body. It gives firmness and elasticity to the skin.

But collagen production decreases with age. You can naturally support the **production of collagen** in your body. Make sure to:

- Sleep well,
- Reduce sugar and tobacco,
- Take vitamin C,

Test: food supplements based on collagen and hyaluronic acid.

3) 4 ways to fight against oxidative stress

Did you know: Wrinkles, Cataract, Emphysema, Cancer, Infarction, Parkinson's disease... More than 100 age-related disorders and diseases are related to free radicals.

While functioning, the cells of our body produce waste: free radicals, responsible for oxidative stress.

You can help the body **fight free radicals** naturally:

- Eat colorful vegetables (for their polyphenols),
- Reduce your stress level (meditation),
- Practice intermittent fasting,
- Fill up on vitamin C and omega 3 and 6

Test: Take food supplements based on vitamins A, C, E, zinc and selenium.

4) Breathe well to live better

Did you know that? The body eliminates 70% of toxins through breathing.

We pay very little attention to how we breathe. **Wrongly so**.

Breathing well allows the body to better eliminate toxins, to have more energy, to have a better quality of sleep, to lose weight and to manage stress.

Abdominal breathing, yawning, holding your breath, cardiac coherence ... are exercises to be practiced daily to take full advantage of the **power of breathing**.

Read more: «Just Breathe: Mastering Breathwork» by Dan Brule and Tony Robbins.

5) Fighting the weight of the years, it's all in the posture

"Confidence is everything, and the way you carry yourself, your posture, eye contact, all of that is such a big role in impressions, regardless of your size."
Camille Kostek, American model

After fifty years, the weight of the years, computers, tablet PCs, make the back bend and the shoulders fall down.

However, good posture is a prerequisite to stay and look younger.

Bodybuilding, stretching, swimming, Nordic walking or even yoga exercises... all help to improve posture.

As a result, you can swagger again and look great.

Do: Practice regular physical activity to keep your back healthy.

6) Joint pain, stiffness, rheumatism... still a question of collagen.

«Drink your broth and don't forget to suck the marrow bone so you don't get sick this winter» Our grandmothers used to say.

Keeping joints healthy requires regular physical activity. Thermal cures can be beneficial.

But preserving and repairing your joint capital after the age of 50 depends above all on diet, especially collagen intake.

Cement of our joints, collagen promotes the formation of cartilage, tendons and ligaments. This protein is found in offal, marrow bones.

Advice: Consume bone broth regularly. More practical, opt for supplementation in Collagen, beef powder protein gelatin.

7) Glutathione to fight Parkinson's, cancers and other age-related degeneration

Did you know that? In 2002, Professor Luc Montagnier (Nobel Prize in Medicine) advised Pope John Paul II to use a mixture of fermented papaya, enriched with Glutathione to treat his advanced form of Parkinson's disease. The pope's health improved greatly immediately afterwards.

Glutathione... behind this barbaric name is a molecule produced naturally by the body. Glutathione is nicknamed the "**master antioxidant**" because it fights oxidative stress.

This oxidation phenomenon is involved in many chronic diseases.

Alas, the production of Glutathione declines with age and makes us more vulnerable to the threats of free radicals. The rusting of our body.

Advice: Glutathione is available in many dietary supplements. Prefer the liposome versions that are better assimilated by the body.

8) Cryotherapy: a few minutes of big chills

*Did you know that? After a few minutes of cryotherapy, the
skin is tighter and the body has consumed
between 800 and 1,200 calories.*

Already, Hippocrates mentioned the benefits of cold to
heal himself.

Today, it is possible to be exposed to abyssal
temperatures in cryotherapy cabins.

Rheumatism, immune system, detox, skin radiance,
aging, better sleep ...

The benefits of cryotherapy are enormous in the fight
against **aging**. Extreme cold allows the body to repair itself,
so that it needs less medication.

Advice: Prefer a cure of 8 to 15 sessions of cryotherapy.
On a smaller scale, you can finish each shower with cold
water. It's already a good start

9) The secret to having more energy: pamper your mitochondria

«Mitochondria support human life because they generate the energy that powers our cells» Sara Adaes, biochemist

The mitochondria are our roommates. They are part of our cells. We compare them to power plants.

Breathing, movement, reflection... work with the energy released by the mitochondria.

At age 50, mitochondria tire and produce less energy.

Caloric restriction, physical exercise, sleeping well, reducing stress, exposure to sunlight and cold ... stimulate mitochondrial optimization.

Read more: «Mitochondria and the Future of Medicine: The Key to Understanding Disease, Chronic Illness, Aging, and Life Itself» by Doctor Lee Know

10) Chronic inflammation, how to fight it with food

«Chronic inflammation, this silent killer, promotes the degeneration of cells and tissues such as joints (osteoarthritis), tendons, muscles, vessel walls (arteriosclerosis)»
extract from the full anti-aging site*

Chronic inflammation affects many people in their fifties. Its symptoms are not very visible. This inflammatory state accelerates aging when it lasts over time.

A healthy diet and a healthy lifestyle combat chronic inflammation. Certain Herbs and Spices are to be consumed regularly to **fight against this inflammatory state**:

- Saffron, cayenne pepper, ginger, cinnamon, cloves, sage, rosemary.

Read more: «The Anti-Inflammatory Diet Protocol: How to Beat Chronic Inflammation, Lose Weight and Heal Your Body With Whole Foods» by Jessica Campbell.

Chapter 11

Couple
10 Tips to strengthen the bonds of the couple at age 50

Couple

«Where better to be than with your family?»
Jean-François Marmontel, French philosopher

At the age of 50, questions about the couple are legion.

What is a happy couple? It is already uncommon, only 15 to 20% of couples are happy in the long term (according to one study).

What is the secret of couples that last? There is no magic formula. Happiness seems to be made of little things and tenderness.

**10 tips to get involved and strengthen
the bonds in your relationship**

1) Take stock of your couple to know where you are going.

«No man has enough memory to succeed in lying.»
Abraham Lincoln, American statesman

After the passion of the beginnings, routine and habits settle in a couple.

It's time for your check-up: Do you still love your partner?
Why are you in a relationship? What are the values of your couple?
Can your relationship evolve?

These are some questions to ask yourself to take stock of your relationship. Should we stop or continue?

Read more: «Couples Therapy Workbook: 30 Guided Conversations to Re-Connect Relationships» by Kathleen Mates-Youngman.

2) Find each other, last, spice up... the 2-2-2 rule for you and your loved one.

«We consider our spouse so much a part of the scenery that we can't think enough about showing our interest in him or her»
Dale Carnegie, American author

Routine often sets in after the wedding. The couple no longer exists, replaced by the family, the children, the dog, the house....

The **2-2-2 rule** suggests that we plan in LOVE and just for us:

- One evening out every 2 weeks,
- One weekend every 2 months,
- One week vacation every 2 years

All face to face, cell phones off.

Do: Take out your agendas. Plan ahead. Book... and get to know each other again.

3) Eating in the evening with your family: strengthens bonds and harmony.

«Half of the interviewees prepare a different dish than the other members of the household, and the blended siblings adapt so as not to offend anyone», says the study.

According to research, the importance of family dinner is declining. Often, everyone eats what they want, when they want and where they want. Yet eating together for a family is crucial.

Like cement, this moment strengthens the bonds of the couple and the family at fifty.

Food choice, regularity, task sharing, conviviality... the evening meal becomes a moment of **harmony**.

Do: Get into the kitchen. Surprise your family by cooking up some good meals, prepared with love.

4) Communicate better in your relationship! Easier said than done

«The most important thing in communication is to hear what is not being said» Peter Drucker, Austrian philosopher

Communicating is essential for the couple's health and self-esteem.

Expressing one's feelings and needs, making clear requests, taking the time to listen, keeping quiet, preferring the "I" to the "You"... are the first steps towards more **intimacy**, **respect** and **love** in the couple.

A peaceful atmosphere is created in the home.

Read more: «The 5 Love Languages: The Secret to Love That Lasts» by Gary Chapman.

5) Do we really want to be involved in our relationship at age 50?

«I'm fed up, I'm the one who takes care of everything in this shack» A common complaint from thousands of women.

What if at age 50, the man would silence this grievance?

The couple is like a fire. It must be fed so that it burns. While taking care of him, taking his health in hand, the quinquagenarian can:

Innovate, propose, cook, invent, think, invest in his couple to strengthen the bonds.

Keeping the Fire Lit In Your Relationship or Marriage

Do: Surprise your wife this week by proposing something new.

6) The couple and happiness... first a question of chemistry

«We find everything in our memory: it is a kind of pharmacy, a chemical laboratory, where we get our hands on a calming drug or a dangerous poison» Marcel Proust, Sodom and Gomorrah

Happiness is above all a chemical process. Four hormones give rise to pleasant sensations and feelings of joy.

Their production in our brain is triggered in several ways:

- **Dopamine**: often say to yourself I've succeeded
- **Endorphin**: laughter, exercise, stretching
- **Oxytocin**: touch, massages
- **Serotonin**: feeling of pride

Read more: «Habits of a Happy Brain: Retrain Your Brain to Boost Your Serotonin, Dopamine, Oxytocin, & Endorphins» by Loretta Graziano Breuning.

7) These 5 little shortcomings that lasting couples don't do

«Excessive jealousy is often the first cause of separation»
Stanislas Leszczynski, King of Poland and Duke of Lorraine

The future of your couple is uncertain, if these situations speak to you:

- Reliving old grudges,
- Do not apologize, do not forgive,
- Blame the other if something is wrong,
- Do not question yourself.

Take advantage of the advice in this guide to reinvent yourself in your fifties. Become a better version of yourself.

Read: "The Sedona Method: Your Key to Lasting Happiness, Success, Peace and Emotional Well-Being" by Hale Dwoskin.

8) Honesty and Sincerity in a couple

«Do not run two hares at the same time» French proverb

Women are endowed with a powerful sixth sense. The secrecy, deceit, and shortcomings of their spouse are felt. And quickly discovered.

Leave no door open to **ambiguous** feelings. Beware of text messages and emails with people of the opposite sex.

A working couple requires Honesty and Control.

Do: testify, cultivate your love for your spouse.

9) Doing things together after 50

«Who looks alike, assembles» French proverb

At age 50, the preoccupations of professional life fade away. For some, the time of retirement is already approaching (the lucky ones).

Give yourself and your family more time. Shared activities (new, old) bring the couple closer together and strengthen them.

Use your imagination. Ask yourself and your spouse about common passions.

Do: cooking, sports, travel, gardening... what activities would you like to share with your partner?

10) Sometimes moving on in a couple is the only solution.

«When two hearts no longer beat in unison, separation is the cure» Julie de Lespinasse, French letter-writer

Undergone or chosen, sometimes the separation comes at the age of fifty. The couple is bled dry, the paths have drifted apart.

Making a successful separation, turning the page, making a clean sweep of the past is far from easy. It leaves traces.

Questioning oneself and having new projects are necessary steps to rebuild oneself.

Read more: «Divorce Recovery: The Ultimate Guide How to Succeed After a Divorce or Separation» by Carolyn Roks.

Chapter 12

Relationship
10 Tips to get what you want after 50 years old

«There are those whom you meet, whom you barely know, who tell you a word, a sentence, give you a minute, a half hour and change the course of your life» Victor Hugo, French writer

How to increase its influence and power of persuasion at the age of 50?

Previous chapters have dealt with health, stress, sleep, food... The chapter "influence and manipulation" focuses on relationships with others.

Friends, family, work... some keys are to be known to be more appreciated and listened to.

***10 tips and techniques to better communicate
and get what you want from others***

1) Stop criticizing and condemning... it's useless.

«You can't teach a man anything, you can only help him to find the answers within himself» Galileo
Italian astronomer and mathematician

You will not change anyone or anything by criticizing.

Criticism is futile and useless. It puts the other person on the defensive, hurts self-esteem and causes resentment.

Try to understand and put yourself in the other person's shoes. Stop making judgments about everything. It is the mark of open, tolerant, more humane minds.

Read more: This advice is the first Dale Carnegie gave in his excellent book «How to Win Friends and Influence People». Written in 1936, this book stays a reference in human relationships.

2) The secret to being instantly loved: Learn the art of complementing people

«Compliments only confirm what we think of ourselves»
Anne Barratin, French writer and philanthropist

This skill requires training, tact and sincerity.

Being attentive to others, noticing and praising a quality, progress, an effort.

To highlight the other person, to boost one's self-esteem. Give **importance** to the other person.

Compliment spontaneously and without ulterior motive to make you loved by all. It is magic.

Do: Be attentive to others. Notice and express a compliment.

3) Take a real interest in others by asking questions.

«Who questions leads» Proverb

Do you want to gain influence and be admired by others?

It's simple. Learn how to ask questions and listen to the answers.

Discover a person's passions, dreams and fears. It's a great way to show them how important they are.

People need recognition and appreciation, the pillars of self-esteem.

Read more: «Doesn't Hurt to Ask: Using the Power of Questions to Communicate, Connect, and Persuade» by Trey Gowdy.

4) Avoid controversy and argumentation

«Looking at people as if they are what they should be, and you
will help them become what they can be»
Goethe, German novelist and poet

You have certainly already attended these deaf people's dialogues where everyone stays on their position. No one listens to anyone, only the will to "nail the other" directs the exchanges.

In these situations, arguing is useless. Express your opinion and listen to those of others. But avoid controversy and change the subject or the person.

Do: develop your listening skills and stop arguing.

5) Donald Trump's secret techniques for persuasion

*«Criticism is easy to take when you realize that those who are
not criticized are the ones who don't take risks»*
Donald Trump, President of the United States

Trump became President of the United States through his skills as a negotiator and speaker.

People are **irrational beings**. Donald Trump plays on emotions, not facts or technical data. He addresses emotional intelligence, speaks simple language, uses short sentences.

He always repeats the same arguments and tells stories to convince.

Read more: «Trump: The Art of the Deal» by Donald Trump.

6) Reciprocity the secret to get from the other what you want

«In politics, citizens solicit favors from politicians who will be returned in the form of votes in elections»
Excerpt from the Toplexis site

Reciprocity is a powerful psychological spring in the human mind. You feel indebted if someone does something for you.

Conversely, to grant a favor to someone, makes the other person feel obliged to return it, for fear of being seen as a profiteer, an ingrate.

Our society is governed by this imaginary contract, by this social norm.

Do: Pay attention, the next time you are offered a coffee, a fruit juice, in a car dealership. You will then be well able to leave with a new car.

7) Social proof reassures and drives to action

*«Today, we use the opinion of others to decide what we buy...
it is the strength of social proof»*

To give more weight to your messages, to what you say, you need to show that other people feel the same way. This is the role of social evidence.

Opinions, recommendations, comments... influence the decisions of those who doubt and don't know what to choose.

Social proof is the best way to convince others to think like you.

Read more: «Methods of Persuasion: How to Use Psychology to Influence Human Behavior» by Nick Kolenda.

8) How do you know if you are being lied to!

Did you know this? A study has shown that 60% of people lie several times during a 10-minute casual conversation.

At fifty, you don't want to be fooled anymore. Some signs do not deceive to detect lies.

Start a discussion by asking trivial questions to study the other person's behavior.

Then move on to more specific questions. The body stiffens, breathing changes... these are signs related to stress.

Giving too many details, vague answers or feigning indignation are all signs that you are being lied to.

Read more: «Unmasking the Face» by Paul Ekman.

9) Giving a good reputation to deserve, the key to inspiring

«Give him a good reputation to justify, and he will make prodigious efforts to avoid demerit in your eyes»
Dale Carnegie, American writer

How do you get the best out of others?

Pointing out: mistakes, flaws and faults have no positive influence on actions and thoughts.

Instead, prefer **beautiful values** and **noble feelings**. Give the other person a good reputation to live up to.

Behave with a person "as if" he or she already has all the qualities you would like him or her to have.

Read more: Reread «how to win friends and influence people» by Dale Carnegie.

10) Showing self-confidence to increase your persuasiveness

«To fly with the eagles, you have to stop swimming with the ducks» T. Harv Eker, American author and businessman

When you have confidence, you naturally look more convincing. Confidence confers authority and credibility.

Whether it is real or fake, playing all the angles makes you feel more confident.

The way you dress, your personality, the way you speak increase your power of persuasion and conviction.

Read more: the book «Unlimited Power» by Tony Robbins.

Chapter 13

Professional
10 Tips to stay
bankable at work
after age 50

«Live as if you had to die tomorrow, learn as if you had to live forever...» Buddha, spiritual leader 6th century BC

The working world is changing, but the way it works remains the same.

Everyone's compensation depends on their level of skill and expertise.

Like a ladder, the more skilled you are, the more value you add.

It's up to each individual to ask themselves what knowledge they need to acquire to increase their market value, whether in their job or by creating their own business.

10 tips to become more efficient and bankable in your fifties

1) How to escape the burnout before switching off

«Burnout is the disease of motivated, committed,
independent, rigorous and combative people»
Annabelle Péclard, work psychologist

Sleep disorders, lack of appetite, extreme fatigue, loss of efficiency, work overload ... burnout awaits you.

5 tips to get out of it:

- Listen to your body, your intuition
- Pause your brain (meditation)
- Don't stay isolated, talk
- Ask for help
- Stop overloading yourself with work, no one will thank you.

Read more: «Burnout to Breakthrough: Building Resilience to Refuel, Recharge, and Reclaim What Matters» by Eileen McDargh.

2) How to break work, sleep, rat race routine?

«To live is to change. This is the lesson that the seasons teach us» Paulo Coelho, Brazilian novelist

If your work is summed up by routine, stress, boredom, hierarchy... it's time to act.

How can you change direction or bounce back after the age of fifty?

- Listening to your instincts for change
- Don't act on a whim, have a plan.
- Changing habits, breaking the routine
- Learn new skills, take action
- Remaining in the position and creating one's own business.

Do: Learn one new skill per term. See the Udemy site (more than 100,000 online courses).

3) 5 steps to request a salary increase

«In the last few months, I've been doing this, this and that. I've brought this, this and that in terms of results...»
Examples of sentences to ask for a raise.

1) Ask for an appointment with his hierarchy.
2) Be in the right timing.
3) Highlight your achievements, the results obtained, the value created... in short, be concrete.
4) Set a range.
5) Have a plan B, a raise is not only about salary.

Finally, on average, by changing employers, the salary increases by 10 to 30%.

Do: Detail precisely the perimeter of your functions and all your accomplishment.

4) The secret to winning a negotiation

«In each of us there is a David and a Goliath»
Robert Kiyosaki, American writer

How to be a good negotiator? Are there techniques, secret strategies to negotiate?

No, life is not like in the movies.

To win a negotiation, you have to be able to give up and leave the table.

Don't rush, prepare yourself before each negotiation. Set yourself limits, a margin, rules and respect them.

Be firm and without regret.

Do: Have a plan B, you'll be even stronger.

5) Multitasking: the really bad idea for productivity

«To be everywhere is to be nowhere»
Seneca, Roman philosopher

The modern world encourages going fast, to do several things at the same time. *Smartphone, computers, e-mail, social media...* allow it easily.

But is it really productive? Studies show it isn't. Multitasking, the **perpetual** change of activity, would make you lose up to 40% of your productivity.

Our brain is not designed for multitasking. Do one thing at a time, but well.

Do: To stay focused on the task at hand, be sure to eliminate outside distractions (notifications, calls...).

6) Speaking in public, take care of the catchphrase to get off to a good start.

Did you know that? For some, the fear of public speaking comes before the fear of death.

Anecdote, riddle, survey, statistics, staging, shock announcement... These six techniques make it possible to start a public speaking by immediately capturing the audience's attention.

Avoid starting your speech with the word "so" or with apologizing or by saying "I'm not a expert, but"

In any case, a good preparation also helps to reduce stage fright.

Learn more: the Toastmasters YouTube channel and videos

7) How to make his writing impactful: The Art of Copywriting

«Copywriting or the art of seducing and convincing an individual to act in the desired direction using simple words»

How to put into words the desire to act: the PAS method (*Problem, Agitate, Solution*) in 3 steps.

1) **Describe** an issue facing your audience,
2) **Shake up** the problem by playing on emotions, describe it to show empathy with the reader,
3) **Present** your solution.

P.A.S. is a powerful framework for building powerful writing.

Read more «On Writing: A Memoir of the Craft Hardcover» by Stephen King.

8) At 50, you can't control everything.

«Give me the serenity to accept the things I cannot change, the courage to change the things I can, and the wisdom to know the difference» The Serenity Prayer

Divorce, dismissal, illness... can occur after the age of fifty.

Blaming it on bad luck or your ex-wife, crying out for injustice won't help you much.

Accept the situation, monopolize your energy to find resources and solutions. Produce the efforts to overcome the ordeal.

You can't control everything. But you remain in control of your reactions.

Do: Get in the habit of knowing what is in your control and what is not. You will gain serenity.

9) How to be more productive, Parkinson's law

«Time is your most faithful ally. Many things can be done in ten minutes...» Ingwar Kamprad, Founder of IKEA

We are not talking about the disease here. We are talking about a law on **self-efficacy**.

According to Parkinson's, each task ends up being spread out over the time allotted to it.

Example with these meetings of 4 hours which is summarized in 1/2 hour of effective work.

Get into the habit of setting deadlines and prefer short work cycles.

Idea: Do like Ingwar Kampra (IKEA founder), who divides his work into short 10-minute periods, even for meetings and phone calls.

10) 4 reasons to start learning English in your 50s

Did you know that: English is the
official language of 75 countries?

Author's note: This book was originally written for French people who are terrible at speaking English. The idea is that it's always good to learn some news skill in your job.

1) Speaking English is one of the skills most in demand by employers.

2) The language of the internet: about 80% of the content on the internet is in English.

3) English is a great way to travel, 3 Billion people speak this language.

4) Learning English (or another language) stimulates memory, develops reasoning and reduces the risk of Alzheimer's, only good things after 50 years old.

Give it a try: Why not listen to English content in your car via podcasts available on Spotify, Deezer?

Chapter 14

Finances
10 Tips to improve your finances and prepare for retirement at the age of 50

«I broke Noah's rule: predicting rain doesn't count. What is important is to build arches» Warren Buffett, American businessman

What do you do when your 50's are knocking on your door and you have neglected your retirement, your finances?

Improving your financial education, making a budget, preparing for retirement... are among the first thing to consider.

And why is it dangerous to depend only on your salary?

Finally, financial serenity comes from being able to enjoy several sources of income.

10 tips to reconsider your finances and prepare for retirement

1) At fifty years of age, you are your greatest resource.

«If a man empties his purse in his head, no one can take it away from him. An investment in knowledge always pays the best interest» Benjamin Franklin, American businessman

Investing is not only limited to the stock market or real estate.

Courses, books, training... the possibilities to acquire new knowledge are numerous: Capitalizing on knowledge.

But it is useless without being healthy.

Maintain and preserve your body, to have more energy and well-being. Body and mind, your greatest asset is you.

Do: What will you learn this month?

2) How to save hundreds of euros every month

«Today people know the price of everything and the value of nothing» Oscar Wilde, Irish writer and poet

How to save money when the end of the month is often difficult?

The answer is in your **account statements**. Review all the causes of expenses:

Subscriptions, fees (bank service, agio), insurance, bills (telephone, electricity, heating), flat rates...

Ask yourself for each expense: **Keep - Delete - Renegotiate**.

You will be surprised by how much money you spend unnecessarily.

Do: Study your bank statements and start to manage your money.

3) Improve your financial education after age 50

*«Money is earned by all those who with patience and
observation go behind those who lose it»*
Benito Pérez Galdos, Spanish novelist

It will not have escaped you, you don't learn how to manage your budget at school.

Understand money, how it works, to make better decisions and control your finances.

Manage your budget, invest, save, start your own business or prepare for retirement,

It is essential to **perfect** your financial education. Books, blogs, courses... there are many ways to learn.

Read more from blogs: «The Simple Dollar» by Trent Hamm or «Money Crashers» by Andrew Schrage and Gyutae Park. The book "All Your Worth: The Ultimate Lifetime Money Plan" Elisabeth Warren

4) Diversifying sources of income at age 50

Did you know that: Millionaires have on average seven different sources of income.

Many people in their fifties have only one source of income: their salary.

This situation has limits that the slightest virus or misfortune can blow out. The solution is to have several sources of income.

- Learn the mechanisms of the stock market (dividends),
- Invest in real estate (rent),
- Build a complementary income in addition to one's work (Side Hustle).

Read more: Side Hustle School by Chris Guillebeau.

5) Side Hustle or how to transform one's passions into sources of income

«What would you do if you weren't afraid?»
Sheryl Sandberg, American businesswoman

The concept of Side Hustle is to use one's passions and skills to create a new source of income. This activity starts in parallel with his job.

The Side Hustle is used to make some extra cash each month, but can possibly replace its salaried activity.

Without risk, the Side Hustle requires a weak financial investment.

Read more: «Side Hustle – From Idea to Income in 27 Days» – Par Chris Guillebeau.

6) How much do you need to save for retirement?

«Old age begins when children retire»
Philippe Bouvard, French journalist and writer

The 4% rule easily gives us the answer. Here's how it works: Estimate the annual amount you will need at retirement and multiply it by 25.

Example: A need of 12,000 euros/year (not including retirement benefits) requires a capital of 300,000 euros.

You will be able to withdraw 4% per year of your capital invested in shares and bonds.

Read more: «The 4% Rule and Safe Withdrawal Rates In Retirement (Financial Freedom for Smart People)» by Todd R. Tresidder .

7) Staying healthy is the best investment

«*Getting up early in the morning and going to bed early are the best rule of thumb to maintain health, money, wealth and good judgment*» *Agricultural proverb*

Health, work, marriage, retirement... you can't control everything in life.

At age 50, however, you may decide to pay more attention to yourself: drink less, quit smoking, work out, eat better, etc.

These **new habits** provide well-being and energy. The essential to start beautiful projects or a new life.

Do: Aim to improve all areas of your life. Don't focus on just one area (*diet, work out...*) to make real changes in your living.

8) Looking for a heavenly retreat? Pack your suitcases

Did you know this? The federal government now sends Social Security checks to 680,000 American retirees who live in other countries, the Social Security Administration reports (boston.com)

The retirement age is a matter of debate and concern. For example, more and more American are considering moving abroad to take advantage of a lower cost of living.

There are many criteria to consider when choosing a country:

Instead of Florida or Arizona, more and more are opting for South or Central America, Mexico, the Caribbean, or Europe... for retirement.

Read more: «Mission: Rescue Your Retirement: How Moving Abroad Saved Our Assets» by Edd Staton

9) Preparing for retirement at age 50, a question of anticipation

«Better late than never» French proverb

Age 50 is probably the last limit to start saving for retirement.

Depending on your risk aversion, choose one or more investments to compensate for the loss of future income.

Life insurance, savings book, stock savings plan... find out more before choosing a solution.

Schedule monthly withdrawals as soon as possible.

Find out more: Subscribe to a financial magazine.

10) How to get rich?

«Wealth is not the amount of money you have but the way you use it» Paulo Coelho, Brazilian writer

Being rich is more than just amounts on a bank statement. It's more about a philosophy.

You can become smarter, more cultured and therefore richer in knowledge.

You can change your behavior and habits to have a fulfilling life.

We become rich by thinking, taking a step back, making plans and taking action.

Do: Learn something new this month.

About the Author

"If you want things to change, You have to change. If you want things to be better, You have to be better." Jim Rohn

Roger. C. Depetris was born in 1968 in the East of France. His 50 years has been marked by an awakening:

The need to regain control of one's health

The writing of this guide required two years of work, research and especially experiments on itself. The author applies most of the advice in this guide.

His health problems (*hypertension, respiratory problems*), which appeared at the age of 40, are much better. He is full of energy and new projects.

Roger lives near Metz (pronounce it like the word mess) where he has been married for more than 20 years.

His wish is to help all new 50-year-olds to create new habits to live better and longer after 50.

More info

avoir50ans.com - avoir50ans@gmail.com

Resources

Chapter 1 - Take Stock of Your Life and Set New Goals

-Ted Talk, video of Josh Kaufman on his book the first 20 hours https://www.youtube.com/watch?v=5MgBikgcWnY

-Summary of Josh Kaufman's book https://des-livres-pour-changer-de-vie.com/les-20-premieres-heures/

-What goals to set in life https://www.penserchanger.com/quels-objectifs-me-fixer-dans-la-vie

-Goals, from the book The Personal MBA https://personalmba.com/goals/

-Objectives according to Steve Pavlina
 https://www.stevepavlina.com/blog/2006/08/how-to-set-goals-you-will-actually-achieve/

-Climbing Everest https://www.20minutes.fr/voyage/2550931-20190627-alpinisme-gravir-everest-quete-ultime-sommet

-Midlife crisis https://www.medecindirect.fr/20190312-crise-de-la-cinquantaine/

-Good or how to be more resilient according to Jocko Willick https://youtu.be/IdTMDpizis8

- 13 steps to be more resilient https://nospensees.fr/13-etapes-developper-resilience/

-13 steps to be more resilient https://medium.com/@lepositifcom/20-des-meilleurs-sites-web-pour-apprendre-quelque-chose-bd5f4f2b3b25

- Article with crazy ideas https://bestlifeonline.com/things-to-do-before-you-die/

-Make a list https://www.passeportsante.net/fr/Actualites/Dossiers/DossierComplexe.aspx?doc=bucket-list-comment-la-creer

Chapter 2 - Combattre le stress –

Le sang plus épais https://www.mapositiveattitude.com/stress/
Les vertus de la méditation
https://www.doctissimo.fr/html/psychologie/stress_angoisse/articles/1
0214-meditation-yoga-vertus-stress.htm#meditation-pour-chasser-le-
stress
Etude norvégienne sur les bienfaits du rire
http://blog.seniorenforme.com/avoir-de-lhumour-fait-augmenter-
votre-esperance-de-vie-de-20/
Comment gérer le stress par le rire https://www.fedecardio.org/Je-m-
informe/J-apprends-a-gerer-mon-stress/prevenir-le-stress-par-le-rire
Vidéo YouTube Exercice de respiration abdominale
https://youtu.be/5tBtaK4fAdA
Le burn out https://www.capital.fr/votre-carriere/burn-out-les-bons-
reflexes-pour-prevenir-et-guerir-l-epuisement-professionnel-1091370
Etude britannique sur notre addiction au portable
https://www.standard.co.uk/news/techandgadgets/average-
smartphone-user-checks-device-221-times-a-day-according-to-
research-9780810.html
Le stress et l'anxiété liés à l'addiction aux smartphones
https://www.numerama.com/tech/345480-nouvelle-etude-lie-lanxiete-
stress-a-laddiction-aux-smartphones.html
La production d'endorphines https://www.personal-sport-
trainer.com/blog/endorphine/
Les endorphines, ces hormones du bonheur
https://magicformlongjumeau.fr/partons-a-la-decouverte-des-
endorphines-ces-hormones-du-bonheur/
Ce besoin de ranger
https://www.vice.com/fr/article/598wn8/pourquoi-faire-le-menage-
destresse-certaines-personnes

Chapter 3 - Sleep, fight the hard nights -

- Les matelas nous empoissonnent -
https://www.consoglobe.com/matelas-substances-toxiques-cg
- Sommeil, voici ce qui arrive si vous ne dormez pas assez
https://www.huffingtonpost.fr/2018/03/16/journee-mondiale-du-
sommeil-voici-ce-qui-arrive-si-vous-ne-dormez-pas-
assez_n_4583755.html
- Temps de sommeil pour les hommes de 50 ans
https://sante.lefigaro.fr/actualite/2015/02/05/23348-combien-dheures-
sommeil-avez-vous-besoin
- Faut-il avoir peur de la lumière bleue?
https://www.francetvinfo.fr/sante/smartphones-tele-tablettes-faut-il-
vraiment-avoir-peur-de-la-lumiere-bleue_2612354.html
- Faire du sport le matin https://sciencenordic.com/denmark-fitness-
sleep/exercise-in-the-morning-and-sleep-better-at-night/1436958
- Un coach en sommeil pour Ronaldo https://www.sofoot.com/un-
coach-de-sommeil-pour-cristiano-ronaldo-205260.html
- Etude sur les bienfaits de la lumière du jour sur le sommeil
https://www.passionsante.be/index.cfm?fuseaction=art&art_id=28461
- Les bienfaits du Groundig https://www.earthing-
vitalite.org/earthing/les-bienfaits-du-earthing-grounding-sur-la-sante-
en-general/
- Les bienfaits du Grounding https://www.earthing-
vitalite.org/earthing/quest-ce-que-le-earthing-aussi-appele-grounding-
ou-connexion-a-la-terre/
- Les bénéfices du Earthing
https://www.lexpress.fr/styles/forme/earthing-la-nouvelle-tendance-
bien-etre-pour-se-reconnecter-a-la-nature_2120279.html
- Le café empêche-t-il de dormir?
https://www.femmeactuelle.fr/sante/sante-pratique/le-cafe-empeche-t-
il-vraiment-de-dormir-est-ce-une-boisson-coup-de-fouet-2081030
- Le noir total est nécessaire à l'endormissement https://www.science-
et-vie.com/corps-et-sante/dormir-dans-le-noir-complet-est-il-
preferable-7446
- Le sexe et le sommeil http://www.i-share.fr/actualite/le-sexe-et-le-
sommeil

- Dossier de l'INSERM sur le sommeil
https://www.inserm.fr/information-en-sante/dossiers-information/sommeil
- Les bienfaits de la sieste de 10 minutes
https://www.passeportsante.net/fr/Actualites/Dossiers/DossierComplexe.aspx?doc=bienfaits-sieste

Chapter 4 - Physical activity -

- Le système lymphatique
https://fr.wikipedia.org/wiki/Syst%C3%A8me_lymphatique
- Les avantages du mini trampoline
https://www.doctissimo.fr/html/forme/fitness/articles/14842-mini-trampoline.htm
- L'origine des kettelbell http://www.blogimperatif.fr/sentrainer-avec-une-kettlebell/
- Les bienfaits de la kettlebell https://www.personal-sport-trainer.com/blog/kettlebell/
- Les bienfaits du sport à l'extérieur
https://www.huffingtonpost.fr/2016/06/03/raisons-faire-sport-exterieur_n_10279920.html
- Le swissball pour avoir un ventre plat
https://conseilsport.decathlon.fr/conseils/5-bonnes-raisons-dutiliser-un-swiss-ball-tp_13168
- Participer à l'Ironman https://www.wts.fr/vieillissement-courir-apres-50-ans/
- Les bienfaits de la course à pied
https://www.runtastic.com/blog/fr/bienfaits-course-a-pied/
- A 50 ans, il vaut mieux courir que marcher
https://sante.lefigaro.fr/actualite/2015/01/05/23223-tout-age-il-vaut-mieux-courir-que-marcher
- Courir lentement favorise les mitochondries https://www.u-trail.com/887courir-lentement/
- Les bienfaits de la douche froide https://www.madaplus.info/Le-saviez-vous-Les-bienfaits-de-la-douche-froide_a7732.html
- Adoptez les attitudes des chasseurs – cueilleurs
https://www.rtbf.be/tendance/bien-etre/sante/detail_adopter-un-mode-de-vie-similaire-a-celui-des-chasseurs-cueilleurs-permettrait-de-rester-en-bonne-sante?id=10124447
- Faire du sport à jeun : le vrai du faux
http://www.athletesdubienetre.fr/sport-a-jeun/

Chapter 5 -Alimentation

- L'alimentation et les maladies chroniques
https://www.inserm.fr/information-en-sante/dossiers-information/nutrition-et-sante
- Livre : Mangeons Vrai - Halte Aux Aliments Ultra Transformés! par le professeur Fardet Anthony
- Podcast du Dr Chatterjee (en anglais) sur l'alimentation et les rythmes biologiques https://www.youtube.com/watch?v=EK7VH6T_2-o
- Prendre une douche intérieure
https://www.chateaudeau.com/blog/pourquoi-boire-un-verre-deau-au-reveil-est-bon-pour-la-sante
- Quel type d'eau choisir http://www.cfaitmaison.com/cru/cru-eau.html
- Quel type d'eau choisir https://www.psychologies.com/Bien-etre/Prevention/Hygiene-de-vie/Articles-et-Dossiers/Sante-Quelle-eau-boire/4L-eau-en-bouteille
- Les aliments frits https://blog.daveasprey.com/dr-cate-shanahan-376/
- Les aliments frits https://www.sante-sur-le-net.com/fuyez-les-aliments-frits/
- Les aliments frits https://amelioretasante.com/5-aliments-donnent-aspect-fatigue/
- Réduire la consommation de viande rouge
http://www.monsieurappert.com/actu/36_5-raisons-de-diminuer-consommation-viande
- Eviter le sucre, vidéo 2 mn du Docteur David Servan Schreiber
https://www.youtube.com/watch?v=on-BTGkXAMg
- Réduire la viande rouge https://sympa-sympa.com/creation-bien-etre/ces-9-signes-nous-indiquent-que-notre-corps-na-pas-pu-digerer-correctement-la-viande-297560/
- Les dangers des produits allégés
https://www.babelio.com/livres/Chardak-Le-light-cest-du-lourd/1041503
- Édulcorants, marketing ou progrès scientifiques?
https://www.passeportsante.net/fr/Actualites/Dossiers/ArticleComplementaire.aspx?doc=edulcorant_phenomene_do

- Etude SU.VI.MAX https://www.lanutrition.fr/bien-dans-sa-sante/les-complements-alimentaires/les-principaux-complements-alimentaires/les-complements-correcteurs-de-l-alimentation/le-magnesium/les-francais-manquent-de-magnesium
- Nutriments de synthèse vs nutriments naturels https://additifs-alimentaires.net/article-nature-vs-synthese.php
- Dr Saldmann sur le jeûne intermittent https://www.europe1.fr/sante/Frederic-Saldmann-vous-pouvez-fabriquer-votre-sante-790778

Chapter 6 - How to start new habits

- Vidéo sur le principe des 5 secondes https://www.youtube.com/watch?v=Ez9_K43TJWk
- Jocko Willink discipline égale liberté https://podcloud.fr/podcast/yoannhamon/episode/82-resume-extreme-ownership-partie-3-discipline-egal-liberte
- Article sur la méthode KonMari https://medium.com/essentiels/la-m%C3%A9thode-konmari-ou-comment-lart-du-rangement-japonais-peut-changer-votre-vie-a2f9006b2159
- Article du magazine Capital, sur apprendre en permanence https://www.capital.fr/votre-carriere/demain-au-boulot-vous-devrez-apprendre-en-permanence-1323578
- L'effet Placebo https://fr.wikipedia.org/wiki/Effet_placebo
- Lorsque l'horloge interne guide nos prescriptions médicales https://www.santemagazine.fr/sante/dossiers/physiologie/chronobiologie-les-bons-rythmes-pour-etre-en-forme-172084

Chapter 7 - Taking care of yourself

- Etude finlandaise sur les bienfaits du sauna https://www.uef.fi/en/-/syyt-saunan-terveyshyotyihin-alkavat-selvita
- Etude du WWF sur les produits chimiques dans notre sang https://www.notre-planete.info/actualites/715-sang_produits_chimiques
- La chimie et les produits de soin https://www.dossierfamilial.com/actualites/des-substances-toxiques-dans-nos-cosmetiques-354277
- Les bienfaits de l'huile de coco https://www.passeportsante.net/fr/Actualites/Dossiers/DossierComplexe.aspx?doc=huile-coco-bienfaits-peau-oragnisme-digestion
- Les méfaits de l'alcool sur la Testostérone https://www.espace-musculation.com/oestrogene.html
- Limiter sa consommation d'alcool https://www.alcoolassistance.net/files/documents/Livret-pour-reduire-sa-consommation.pdf
- Les mauvais effets des lunettes de soleil https://themodelhealthshow.com/side-effects-of-sunglasses/
- Les bénéfices de la douche froide https://www.msn.com/en-us/health/health-news/12-benefits-of-taking-cold-showers-every-day/ar-BBUq4zD
- Les bains froids en Finlande:https://finland.fi/fr/vie-amp-societe/le-plongeon-hivernal-frais-devant/
- Adoptez la bonne position https://blog.vivre-mieux.com/sante-bien-etre/readoptez-une-position-naturelle-aux-toilettes/
- Le squatty potty https://www.amazon.fr/Squatty-Potty-constipation-daffaiblissement-dincontinence/dp/B007BISCT0
- L'intestin, notre deuxième cerveau https://www.doctissimo.fr/sante/atlas-corps-humain/question-corps-humain/intestin-deuxieme-cerveau

Chapter 8 - Health, threats hover over the new quinqua

- Les maladies liées au mode de vie
https://fr.wikipedia.org/wiki/Maladie_li%C3%A9e_au_mode_de_vie
- Pourquoi réaliser les bilans sanguins et cardiaques
https://www.allodocteurs.fr/actualite-sante--ans-l-heure-du-bilan_11783.html
- Mesurer ses taux hormonaux
https://www.thierrysouccar.com/sante/info/hommes-5-examens-indispensables-50-ans-2297
- 1 personne sur 30 touchée par le cancer colorectal
https://www.frm.org/recherches-cancers/cancer-du-colon/quelques-chiffres-sur-le-cancer-colorectal
- 18 000 décès dus au cancer colorectal
https://www.santepubliquefrance.fr/presse/2018/cancer-colorectal-18-000-deces-par-an
- Comment garder son cerveau en bonne santé https://www.partena-ziekenfonds.be/fr/magazine/vivre-sainement/voici-comment-conserver-un-cerveau-en-bonne-sante
- Comment garder son cerveau en bonne santé 2
https://www.santemagazine.fr/sante/maladies/maladies-neurologiques/pour-rester-jeune-prenez-soin-de-votre-cerveau-174398
- Les traitements antihypertenseurs
https://www.santemagazine.fr/traitement/medicaments/quels-medicaments-pour-traiter-une-hypertension-427379
- L'hypertension touche 1 adulte sur 3 https://www.cardio-online.fr/Actualites/Depeches/La-prevalence-de-l-hypertension-arterielle-en-France-n-a-pas-baisse-depuis-2006
- Dysfonction érectile: des exercices plutôt que le Viagra!
https://www.passeportsante.net/fr/Actualites/Nouvelles/Fiche.aspx?doc=2005101159
- La baisse de la testostérone, nos origines
https://www.pourquoidocteur.fr/Articles/Question-d-actu/7445-La-baisse-de-testosterone-serait-a-l-origine-de-la-civilisation-humaine
- Augmenter son taux de testostérone
https://naturalathleteclub.com/blog/augmenter-taux-testosterone/

- Prendre soin de sa prostate (vidéo)
https://www.youtube.com/watch?v=KBmoz05remY
- Comprendre l'importance des rythmes circadiens, l'INSERM
https://www.inserm.fr/information-en-sante/dossiers-information/chronobiologie
- Les maladies chroniques sont en hausse
https://www.lefigaro.fr/conjoncture/2016/12/14/20002-20161214ARTFIG00089-plus-de-10-millions-de-francais-souffrent-d-une-maladie-chronique.php
- Les travaux du professeur Satchin Panda
https://www.medisite.fr/bien-manger-manger-sur-10-heures-le-secret-pour-etre-en-bonne-sante.5490847.72.html
- Les travaux du professeur Satchin Panda 2
https://blog.santelog.com/2018/02/12/horloge-biologique-cest-toute-la-rythmique-de-notre-expression-genique/
- Quand prendre les médicaments
https://www.santemagazine.fr/sante/dossiers/physiologie/chronobiologie-les-bons-rythmes-pour-etre-en-forme-172084
- Les troubles de la vue augmentent
https://www.consoglobe.com/proteger-vue-ecrans-cg

Chapter 9 - Sex and the 50-year-old man -

- Les 4 conséquences du déficit en Testostérone (vidéo de 6mn)
https://youtu.be/sQM2kiBs4YM
- L'andropause https://www.charles.co/blog/sexualite/andropause/
- Le foie un organe extraordinaire https://badgut.org/centre-information/sujets-de-a-a-z/le-foie-un-organe-extraordinaire/?lang=fr
- Le cholestérol et la Testostérone
http://hupnvs.aphp.fr/nutritionbichat/le-cholesterol/
- Jed Diamond https://www.webmd.com/jed-diamond
- L'alcool favorise les œstrogènes chez l'homme
https://www.antiageintegral.com/anti-age-revitalisation/exces-oestrogenes-homme
- L'aromatase https://www.toutelanutrition.com/wikifit/sante/bien-etre/qu-est-ce-que-l-aromatase
- La Testostérone, PDF de Bayer
https://www.bayer.ch/static/documents/Maennergesundheit-FR.pdf
- Faible taux de Testostérone et obésité
https://www.lesupplements.com/fr/base-de-connaissances/articles-de-sante/54-faible-taux-de-testosterone-favorise-l-obesite-abdominale-chez-les-hommes-vieillissants.html
- Sommeil et Testostérone
https://fr.myprotein.com/thezone/lifestyle/baisse-votre-taux-testosterone-causes-traitements/
- Stress et Testostérone
https://fr.myprotein.com/thezone/lifestyle/baisse-votre-taux-testosterone-causes-traitements/
- 10 aliments qui sont mauvais pour la testostérone
https://www.heliopurtech.com/10-aliments-qui-reduisent-la-testosterone/
- Les meilleures sources de lipides
https://www.toutelanutrition.com/wikifit/outils/nutrition/les-meilleures-sources-de-lipides-pour-booster-la-testosterone
- S'orienter vers une alimentation, type paléo
https://www.lanutrition.fr/interviews/thierry-hertoghe-l-un-regime-pauvre-en-cereales-et-laitages-pour-reequilibrer-les-hormones-r

- Supporter son taux de Testostérone par le sport
http://www.enpleinelucarne.net/pratique-du-sport-comment-augmenter-son-taux-de-testosterone/
- Les perturbateurs endocriniens
https://www.perturbateurendocrinien.fr/essentiel/
- Le soleil favorise la Testostérone
https://naturalathleteclub.com/blog/augmenter-taux-testosterone/

Chapter 10 - Aging

- Le site antiageintegral https://www.antiageintegral.com/anti-age-revitalisation/rajeunir-en-douceur
- Le cerveau, privilégiez le gras http://sante.lefigaro.fr/actualite/2015/12/18/24417-pourquoi-il-ne-faut-pas-priver-son-cerveau-gras
- Les bienfaits de la respiration https://www.bloomingyou.fr/bien-respirer-transformer-corps/
- Vidéo 2 mn pour comprendre le rôle des omégas 3 https://www.passeportsante.net/fr/Solutions/PlantesSupplements/Fiche.aspx?doc=acides_gras_essentiels_ps
- Maladies liées au stress oxydatif https://www.santemagazine.fr/alimentation/nutriments/antioxydants/luttez-contre-le-stress-oxydatif-171714
- Compléments alimentaires pour lutter contre le stress oxydatif https://www.fleurancenature.fr/blog/comment-lutter-contre-stress-oxydatif
- Les bienfaits du bouillon de bœuf https://www.remedes-de-grand-mere.com/17-vertus-du-bouillon-dos-et-comment-le-preparer/
- Papaye fermentée et Glutathion https://www.alternativesante.fr/parkinson/pourquoi-diable-le-pape-a-t-il-pris-de-la-papaye
- Le rôle méconnu du Glutathion https://www.alternativesante.fr/glutathion/le-seul-antioxydant-dont-on-ne-nous-parle-jamais
- Article du journal VSD sur les bienfaits de la Cryothérapie https://www.cryojetsystem-france.fr/img/cmsadvanced/pdf/article-vsd-cryotherapie.pdf
- Inflammation chronique et vieillissement https://www.antiageintegral.com/anti-aging/inflammation-chronique-accelere-vieillissement

Chapter 11 - The couple, living well together after turning 50 -

- Etude IFOP sur les repas en famille
https://food.konbini.com/news/les-francais-passent-de-moins-en-moins-de-temps-a-table-le-soir
- 9 bienfaits de manger en famille https://www.goodnet.org/articles/9-scientifically-proven-reasons-to-eat-dinner-as-family
- Les 4 hormones du bonheur https://xn--matransformationintrieure-tic.fr/hormones-du-bonheur/

Chapter 12 - Influence and Manipulation, Little Secrets to Getting What You Want –

- Les techniques de persuasion de Donald Trump
https://www.inc.com/peter-economy/the-6-persuasion-secrets-of-donald-trump-according-to-dilbert-s-scott-adams.html
- Le principe de réciprocité en politique http://www.toplexis.com/non-classe/qui-donne-recoit-le-principe-de-reciprocite-sous-la-loupe-de-robert-cialdini/
- Le principe de réciprocité
https://daniloduchesnes.com/blog/principes-persuasion-robert-cialdini/
- La force de la preuve sociale https://fr.lightspeedhq.com/blog/le-marketing-par-preuve-sociale/
- Savoir reconnaître les mensonges:https://www.huffingtonpost.fr/dr-travis-bradberry/8-signes-qui-montrent-que-lon-vous-ment_a_22118784/

Chapter 13 - Professional, how to overcome the dangerous course of the half-century

- Phrases magiques pour demander une augmentation
https://www.bibamagazine.fr/lifestyle/travail/5-phrases-presque-magiques-pour-demander-une-augmentation-40134.html
- Le site de Pascal Haumont pour s'exprimer facilement en public
https://www.pascalhaumont.fr/
- Les dangers du Multi taches
https://matthieudesroches.com/articles/verite-sur-multitasking-1
- Loi de Parkinson, efficacité et gestion du temps https://www.journee-efficace.fr/loi-de-parkinson/
- 10 choses à savoir sur Ingvar Kamprad
https://www.lefrontal.com/10-choses-a-savoir-a-propos-de-ingvar-kamprad-le-fondateur-d-ikea
- Ressources et idées pour bâtir un SideHustle (site en français)
https://sidehustlefrance.com/

Chapter 14 - Retirement, preparing for and anticipating retirement

- Economisez des centaines d'euros par mois (source en anglais) https://www.iwillteachyoutoberich.com/save-1000-in-30-days-challenge/
- Blog esprit riche https://esprit-riche.com/
- Blog le petit actionnaire https://petit-actionnaire.fr/
- Les gens riches ont 7 sources de revenus https://www.journaldemontreal.com/2016/07/25/les-7-sources-de-revenus-du-millionnaire
- Résumé du livre "Side Hustle – From Idea to Income in 27 Days" https://des-livres-pour-changer-de-vie.com/revenu-complementaire-side-hustle/
- Blog Fin de la Rat Race https://fin-de-la-rat-race.com/
- Page Facebook Side Hustle France https://www.facebook.com/groups/481293465579564/
- La règle des 4% https://monsieurmoneymoustache.com/tag/regle-des-4/
- La retraite à l'étranger https://lepetitjournal.com/expat-pratique/les-paradis-de-retraite-letranger-253504
- Le site Retraite sans frontières http://www.retraitesansfrontieres.fr/

Printed in Great Britain
by Amazon